'As an individual working i   *Circle Holding* was a transformational   ophies and real-time practices that offered light bulb moments in thinking about shared listening and speaking spaces. In the exploration of meaningful connection, the authors' heartfelt voices were especially moving as they led us to gain intimate insight into how various communities engage with the shared values of inclusivity, personal and communal growth. I rode the wave of this book with barely a pause, and I came out the other end with a more visceral understanding of what deeply considered compassionate care can look like.'

       – Shoshana Perry, Narrative 4 Story Exchange facilitator and mindfulness educator

'A gorgeously nourishing book that will open the heart of anyone who reads it. Julia Davis and Tessa Sanderson take us on an inspiring journey, immersing us in knowledge and courage so we know how to design beautiful, inclusive, safe and creative circles in an infinite number of ways.'

       – Fiona Agombar, yoga therapist, author and rest activist

'Julia Davis and Tessa Sanderson have written a well-researched, clearly communicated and compelling story into the art and craft of how important talking circles are and how they work. It is strong theoretically AND practically. This is an essential read for anyone who works in the wellness industry - yoga teacher, Reiki master, sound healer, breathwork facilitator - because all of this work essentially takes place in the sacred space of a circle. I cannot recommend this highly enough.'

       – Benedict Beaumont, Founder of Breathing Space

'A much-needed guide to the art and the skills of circle holding, this book is inviting, accessible and full of inspiration and practical advice. If you work with groups, or you would like to, put it at the top of your reading list - you won't regret it.'

       – Jess Glenny, somatic movement teacher, facilitator, therapist

'Julia Davis and Tessa Sanderson take us gently by the hand and invite us to dive into the possibilities for connection and healing that are calling us to hold space for our communities. Deeply practical, it offers step-by-step guidance on everything we need to consider: who to invite, inclusion, venues and online meetings, preparing the space, marketing, support and money are all laid out. An absolute gem, I wish this book had existed before I held circles – it would have saved me heaps of time, energy and heartache.'

– Kate Codrington, author of *Second Spring* and
The Perimenopause Journal

'Just wow!! This book is ALL THE THINGS when considering or creating a circle. So many authors on this subject focus only on what will be happening during the event, but these authors cover not only those essentials with great passion, insight and depth but then also speak to the "dream space" that will lead you to create a deeply authentic-to-you, congruent and meaningful offering. They then double down on the value by walking the reader step by step through all the technical, logistic, administrative challenges of circle creation by sharing their personal insights and "time in the trenches". It's beautiful, powerful and pretty ESSENTIAL if you'd like to either start your journey creating circles or want to seriously hone your craft!'

– Jenny Burrell, Founder of Burrell Education

'Julia Davis and Tessa Sanderson's clear, approachable discussion of the dynamic process of circle holding in talking circles is vital reading for anyone interested in fostering empathy and empowering positive change. It will be extremely useful for my own work in interfaith and cross-communal conversations. This is a book that will help build the supportive communities of the future and enable anyone to access the necessary skills required to set up and run a circle, enabling us to appreciate and overcome any challenges along the way. It is written with warmth, insight and humour. A significant contribution to changing the culture and building a better society.'

– Ariel Kahn, novelist and associate artist at
the Woolf Interfaith Institute

Circle Holding

CIRCLE HOLDING

A Practical Guide to Facilitating Talking Circles

Julia Davis and Tessa Venuti Sanderson

Illustrations by Tessa Venuti Sanderson

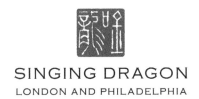

SINGING DRAGON
LONDON AND PHILADELPHIA

First published in Great Britain in 2025 by Singing Dragon,
an imprint of Jessica Kingsley Publishers
Part of John Murray Press

1

A CIP catalogue record for this title is available from the
British Library and the Library of Congress

ISBN 978 1 80501 315 0
eISBN 978 1 80501 316 7

Printed and bound by CPI Group (UK) Ltd, Croydon, CR0 4YY

Jessica Kingsley Publishers' policy is to use papers that are natural,
renewable and recyclable products and made from wood grown in
sustainable forests. The logging and manufacturing processes are expected
to conform to the environmental regulations of the country of origin.

Singing Dragon
Carmelite House
50 Victoria Embankment
London EC4Y 0DZ

www.singingdragon.com

John Murray Press
Part of Hodder & Stoughton Limited
An Hachette UK Company

*In memory of David Shaw who created circles
for family, friends and community. Julia*

*To all those who've sat in circle with me.
The connection lives on. Tessa*

Contents

An invitation

Everything we share in this book is an invitation. Please feel free to take what you find valuable and leave what does not serve your purpose.

Note to the reader: The circle stories and people in this book

We are hugely grateful to the many circle holders who have contributed their knowledge, experience and circle stories through interviews. Many have brought tears to our eyes and laughter to our lips: some of the emotions that can be experienced in circles themselves.

Contributors have chosen whether their full name, first name or a pseudonym appears after a quotation. Some established facilitators have chosen to add their circle name too. All of these people have granted us permission to use their experiences as teaching tools. We share many circle stories in this book. Where they are based on real experience of a specific circle, we will say so. Throughout the book we also share exercises with circles which are a fictionalised mix of different experiences from a variety of circle holders. Any resemblance to real circle holders and real participants is just that.

Introduction

The power of circle

In school we are taught to debate. Importance is placed on having the ability to win an argument. We are also taught how to sit down in silence and listen to a figure of authority. To only speak when spoken to, to put our hand in the air if we want to speak or be picked upon to speak if requested to by a teacher. Our basic needs – for example, to go to the toilet if we have our period – are questioned.

At the dinner table, if we ever sit with others to eat dinner, we probably talk over each other and interrupt. We are offered daily examples in the media of politicians braying at each other and shaming others' views.

Circle provides a different way. A space for us to know that our voices can be heard without ridicule or risk of violence. Somewhere we are given the opportunity to learn listening skills. We have often wondered what the world would look like if these skills were exalted and taught. And in this book we share many examples of where these skills are used in circle gatherings to transform lives.

How to use this book

First things first. A VERY WARM WELCOME.

We are so glad you found your way here and that you're interested in holding circles. Why don't you get a drink and find somewhere really comfortable to sit?

What is a circle and why use one?

If you are interested in creating a space where each person has the opportunity both to speak and be listened to without interruption or comment, then you have come to the right place. This interest often comes from a very specific need and necessitates a gathering of a particular demographic. Circles build connection and community.

We will look at how to facilitate circles of different sizes and manifestations, both in person and online, across many intersections, some of which celebrate intergenerational and cultural connection and others which are designed to suit a very specific demographic. It may be surprising how well many of the precepts shared in this book cross divides and work with widely different groups.

A *practical guide book*

Each chapter has guidance on an aspect of facilitating a circle, stories and exercises. We encourage you to gain inspiration from the stories of different circles around the globe and use the exercises to more clearly shape how you want to hold your circle. If you are thinking of running a circle with colleagues and friends, you may wish to work through them together.

This book has grown out of our love of facilitating circles.

We know our knowledge and experience only goes so far, and that is why research for this book included interviewing a huge range of circle holders with diverse characteristics. We will answer questions about the purpose of listening circles, how we hold space, creating boundaries, time management and responding to red flag situations (and much more) from the combined perspectives of many circle holders and not simply our own.

This book is a collaboration. One thing we have learned along the way is that whether we are running circles alone or with others, we could not have sustained the circles we run without the support of friends, family and colleagues, whether that is someone at home putting dinner on the table or a kind caretaker opening up a venue half an hour in advance to allow for preparation time or a mentor providing feedback on our experiences of circle holding. It takes a village to create a circle!

Talking circles offer a world of possibilities. We aim to bring creativity to what the gathering can be while sharing a clear understanding of structures and frameworks that have been proven to work. Our intention is for you to learn from the mistakes we and others have made so you gain understanding and confidence, and above all a willingness to try, knowing that the journey is often the most exciting and exhilarating part of the process.

It is our wish that you take this work out into your own circles. Reading a book can only take you so far; be brave and put what you learn into action. You might even wish for the purpose of your next circle to be to gather others with the same intention so you can work through this book together!

Guiding you through every aspect of circle holding

The idea of running a talking or listening circle may at first sound easy. A circle is formed. The choice is made for talking to occur without interruption, and each person is given the time and space to speak. And yet there is much more to a circle than you might think. It is possible through skilled facilitation to create space for transformational experience. It is our intention that through using this book you will find answers to the questions:

- Why do you want to form a circle?

- Who is it for?

- How are you going to invite people in?

- What precepts may help the flow of the circle?

- What themes will you use?

- How will you introduce those themes?

- How will the circle open and close?

- What are the practical aspects of circle holding, including timing and location?

Now let's start with what a circle is and is not…

CHAPTER 1

What Is a Talking and Listening Circle?

You're having dinner in a group of people and it's impossible to hear the person next to you, let alone the other people speaking. You don't even try to speak. Your mind starts to drift and you switch off. You dream of a different kind of space where each person is heard fully. Whether you're simply curious about talking circles, have attended or have facilitated them, you might be wondering how to define exactly what a talking circle is and also how to describe what it is not. Is it helpful to talk about creating a safe space? What is 'holding'? In this chapter, we aim to give you an overview of the concept of a talking circle.

This chapter is in two parts: reflecting on the concept of a circle, and providing an overview of what a circle structure might look like. More details on the different components will be given in the following chapters. You will also find chapters on business and marketing, running circles online and a discussion about charging.

What is a talking and listening circle?

In this book, we have used both the terms 'listening circle' and 'talking circle'. Both activities happen in circle time and it is entirely up to you which you put more emphasis on. It is also common to see 'circle' used without these terms, as in women's circle, teens' circle or men's circle, with an implicit understanding that listening and talking will be a component.

By using these terms, you are signalling that a different kind of communication is expected than normally happens in everyday Western life. This communication is based on one person speaking at a time, on the principle that everyone is valued and enabled to talk, and on the understanding that the aim is to listen fully and wholeheartedly. The guiding principles may vary from circle to circle and may include respect, non-judgement, confidentiality, commitment to inclusion and self-responsibility. These will be unpacked further in Chapter 8.

> A circle is a listening space where you listen with all your heart and respect, with an openness to be in a safe space. It's about letting go of planning what to say and giving all of your attention. It's a room with no interruption. It's about confidentiality and trying not to judge (at least out loud!).
>
> *Mandy Lau*

In its purest expression, a listening or talking circle is not group therapy, but it may be cathartic and therapeutic to share with others. It is not a teaching space, where one person is the expert, but you may learn something about yourself or life while attending one. It is not a purely social gathering, but you may socialise as part of it. It is not a solution-focused activity, but may lead to finding answers. However, circles are used within therapy programmes (like Alcoholics Anonymous), within training courses and workshops, and at retreats and festivals and in conflict resolution.

One way we like to conceptualise circle time is as a pressure valve. In society, having a space where people can have their voice heard and considered is paramount for social cohesion. Within people's personal lives, with the inevitable ups and downs, it also provides a function of taking the pressure off one person to cope with and figure out everything on their own.

A circle provides a physical and psychological container for a place to listen with respect to others and for others to listen with respect to you.

What is a safe space?

> The comment that I absolutely love to receive above anything else is when someone says I felt safe. I felt safe to explore, I felt safe to let go, whatever it is, but I felt really safe.

> The most important thing from the beginning is creating that container of safety. You can't guarantee that someone is going to feel safe. We don't have control over that.

At best we can create a container that feels safe enough for someone.

Sophie Cleere

There are ways to create a space in which someone can be reasonably confident that they won't be exposed to criticism, discrimination or harassment, or any other type of emotional or physical harm. This is a fundamental aim to have when facilitating circles. Depending on someone's previous life experiences, going into a new circle may make them feel vulnerable and unsafe by default.

Although we cannot guarantee that our spaces will feel safe for every participant, we can put structures in place with this intention. Communicating that your circle is somewhere participants could feel comfortable starts with the communication about the event, how you welcome them into the space, the outlining of the principles by which the circle runs and listening to feedback.

The term 'safe space' has perhaps become overused and it is impossible to guarantee that you can always provide it. For someone who has experienced trauma, it can be difficult to predict what might be triggering. Another term that we like is 'brave space', which aims to create an environment where an attendee feels comfortable enough to share their authentic experience even when this goes hand in hand with being vulnerable.

> You have to try things. You have to rub up against discomfort because that is where we learn. I don't believe there are any guarantees. You can create a brave space, that's what we want to create, more of that, but there are no guarantees about safety.

Lee Keylock, Director of Global Programs, Narrative 4

An important activity that we share in Chapter 7 is to include a settling practice near the beginning of the circle, to settle everyone's nervous systems after arriving. In Chapter 8, we describe how to create as strong as possible a container through sharing guidelines for communication and behaviour. We want you to feel confident to create these important spaces.

What is holding space?

A term that you may hear people use in relation to circles and counselling is 'holding space'. This may seem paradoxical as you can't physically hold space in your hands, but the concept is about creating a pause in everyday life. This might be difficult to do yourself when there is laundry to be done or emails to be answered. However, when someone else is sitting with you (in person or virtually), giving you their attention, it is easier to stay with that pause and see what comes up.

A key aspect of holding space is that you make the intention for yourself to keep a distance from the person sharing. There is no responsibility to take on emotionally what is shared. It is the responsibility of those in circle to listen without judgement but not to fix or find solutions. As what is shared in circle can be significant and intense, it is important to take this on board. Otherwise, the experience of being in circle as a listener can become overwhelming.

> It isn't just a chit-chat, but a space to be yourself: whatever you are that day, whether to be strong or fall apart. It's a different kind of environment to go inwards. You might not have that space normally depending on your situation, like if you have children or are a carer. In the circle, you don't have to be fixed, you are heard. I've always felt nourished in that space.
>
> *Barbara-Lee*

By being a circle holder, you are creating a space for a group of people to pause. When big emotions arise, you keep holding the emotional environment you've created so that they can be expressed and start to be processed. You are also maintaining the principles that were agreed at the beginning of the circle by reminding people to be kind in their communication.

It is possible for big issues to be addressed in circle time if the container being held allows for this. The facilitator has responsibility for how the container is created and responding to the needs within the group, but ultimately the circle holder is not responsible for the emotional wellbeing of participants: the responsibility for one's wellbeing is in the hands of each participant. A clear guideline of circle holding is: You are responsible for your own wellbeing. Do what you need to do to look after yourself in this space.

As Sophie Cleere puts it, 'Though we can create a space that is as safe as it can be, we have to trust that people can take care of themselves in that space.'

A space in which each person is responsible for themselves and there is no fixing is a container which can feel comfortable. It can be very freeing to know that someone else is not here to solve your problems – the responsibility of those in circle is to act as witness. This is a key difference between circle holding and counselling or therapy.

When starting out with circle holding, a guiding principle is to encourage people to share something small rather than big: a 3–4 out of 10 rather than a 9 out of 10. Then it is less likely that sharing will involve something the circle holder and participants feel uncomfortable listening to. We will share more tips on managing the dynamics of the group in Chapter 7. Time boundaries are also important, and we will look in more depth at how to manage time in Chapter 8.

We are both yoga teachers and so also hold space in that context too. So often, it's only when someone comes into the yoga class and pauses in a position or rests for relaxation that they realise how truly tired they are or have time to face an emotion that's been in the background. In the modern world, it can be easier to rush from activity to activity or numb out through scrolling than to be with the emotions just below the surface. Providing circle time allows people to have space to connect with what is happening for them and have their experiences acknowledged.

> My biggest worries are a fear of responsibility for people's emotions, not being able to handle what may come up. I realise the importance of looking after my own emotional health so that I can help serve others to the best of my ability. I may need more confidence in establishing clear boundaries.
>
> *Brenda Rock*

What is the format of a circle?

There is a basic structure to a listening circle, but many activities that can be added in to support the listening and enrich the experience. The basic structure, circle principles and the additional activities will be expanded upon in the following chapters.

The basic structure is:

- preparation
- welcoming
- opening the circle and settling
- introductions
- framing the circle (principles, what will happen, timing)

- talking/listening

- integration and closing.

Woven into the basic structure may be:

- listening partnerships – speaking to one other person rather than the whole group

- settling practices like meditation, mindful movement

- craft activities – shifting the focus

- ritual and ceremony

- personal reflection time, such as through journalling

- social time – for chatting.

It can be helpful as the circle holder to have a strong sense of timings, structure and themes. Your agenda is likely to look different to what you share with the participants due to your responsibility for timing. Ideally, the length of the circle will be honoured while the participants do not need to hold tightly to the structure of the gathering.

A circle can be elaborate, with ceremony and ritual weaved through different parts of the event.

> I love the ritual and ceremony. I like looking into the fire. Circle for me is about creating a container with a clear sense of intention. Including ritual and ceremony is like going through a portal to somewhere you feel safe. For people whose lives are hectic, a circle is a chance to step away from that and come out feeling revitalised.
>
> *Kate Forde*

There are also circumstances in which talking and listening circles can be very lightly held. If a fire is lit on an evening and a circle forms around it, deep conversations can occur without a need to hold on to structure or strong codes. However, even in these circumstances it can be helpful to have some guidelines.

> There are times when it can feel really effortless. You give people something and the space opens up for them to share their experience. I can sit...and watch the magic happen.
>
> *Kate Codrington, menopause mentor and circle facilitator*

There was a format, it felt safe, people could share what they wanted. There was a flow and a structure, and they were well contained.

Lisa Horwell

Do I need to use the term 'circle'?

No! It is important to be clear about what your intention is when holding space, but you do not have to use the term 'circle' if you think it would be unclear or off-putting for your intended participants. Perhaps the circle element is a small part of what you are offering during a bigger event and there isn't space in your marketing to explain exactly what a circle is and isn't. After all, it's taken a whole chapter to explain it here!

Let's hear more about the magic of circles in the next chapter.

CHAPTER 2

The Magic of Circle Time

Take a moment to imagine a place where you feel comfortable to be yourself and even brave enough to share what makes you feel vulnerable. As you sit with the others in the circle, you feel yourself settling and unwinding. There may be moments where you're on the edge of your seat, feeling awkward about how to respond, in tears, laughing out loud... All of this is held in a container created by the circle holder. In this chapter, we introduce you to the magic of being in a talking circle.

Sitting in circle is an ancient practice. Ever since humans learnt how to create fire, our ancestors have sat in circle. While community spaces exist where people can share their authentic selves, many others do not have this opportunity.

What would the world be like if every person had the opportunity to be listened to in circle and share from the heart on a regular basis? If all our places of learning and working had circle time at their heart? If every life threshold was honoured in circle gatherings and the major life challenges were recognised and listened to? In this chapter, we share the magic of circle time before diving into the practical guidance.

Our vision is to bring circle facilitation into widespread use and hope that you are inspired by the transformational effect of leading circles from the stories in this book. Israh Goodall, a circle holder, shares: 'There is something around circle that just reminds us that every single person that you meet, every single person that sits down, has a unique gift. It provides a space to learn from each other.'

Time and again we have seen the positive and life-affirming changes that can happen through the simple act of speaking without judgement and listening without the need to respond. The experience of being witnessed in circle, whether it is in a one-off gathering or over time in a regular event, can be profound. Before we get into the specifics of facilitating, let's hear from other circle holders about the magic of being in circle...

> It was the authenticity and the true nature of the women that showed up [in circle] that was so compelling.
>
> *Suzan Nolan, Gather the Women*

> The circle represents connection with others. It is something which comes from sharing space with other humans in a ritualised setting.
>
> *Henika Patel*

> The overwhelming sense of peace and calm and meditation when I left the circle is what keeps sending me back every time.
>
> *Anouska Ornstein*

> The structure of circle is useful to break the usual social norms. You can share anything. You feel freer to really express yourself because you know it won't be commented upon.
>
> *Mark Walsh*

We also asked people who attend talking and listening circles to share what the experience means to them:

> Being part of a circle meant I could address feeling vulnerable and sharing a part of me that I'd kept safely closed away. It meant I could learn to be open and to know that what I shared wasn't going to be openly judged; it also meant that I learned the power of challenging the idea and not the person, in a safe and compassionate way.

> My time in circle is cherished and valued and I recognise how much I look forward to belonging to such a special group. The friendships that I have made from being part of the circle have been affirming and enhancing. Being truly heard and seen still feels like a rare and precious treat.
>
> *Joanna Feast*

The next person was curious, but hadn't thought circle gatherings would be for her:

> I initially came to the women's circle out of curiosity and was not expecting to stay. Several years later and I am still here! The circle called to me in a way other social groups did not. Holding my space in a circle of women

was a unique experience for me. There was no male presence or views, which was refreshing and somewhat liberating.

The listening (no fixing) and trust within the circle enabled me to examine and challenge unhelpful childhood beliefs which had been generated by the topics covered and my own self-awareness. In being held by the circle, I have allowed myself to become vulnerable and have felt a softening and a sense of letting go in the process. The power of listening compassionately to each other and the validation that it gives is a special experience each time we meet.

Alison Butler

This man attended an embodied yoga circle:

Often being the only man in the circle has given me a privileged insight into the ways women are seeking to embody their yoga practice. It has helped me reframe my own challenges with greater empathy for others and a better self-understanding.

Ariel Kahn

Sometimes circles meet for a specific reason, such as this one: 'It was a lovely peaceful room: so calm and it felt good to be able to talk openly about perimenopause without judgement' (perimenopause yoga circle attendee).

In our work we often hear from participants who have experienced the magic of being in circle time. It is our intention in this book to share tools you can use to bring about experiences like those described below:

I remember feeling so accepted and free in my first circle. Others were vulnerable which helped me to open up after first feeling anxious about doing so. I remember feeling a strong sense of community and connection that I don't often get elsewhere and that is what brought me back. I recall one women's circle where I couldn't even really describe what we did or why it was special but I felt such a connection that stays with me to this day.

Lydia Martin

CIRCLE STORY: THE MAGIC OF ARRIVING
Julia remembers...

The morning of the circle has arrived. I have prepared. The studio looks lovely. There is a blanket laid down in the centre with oracle cards representing the maiden, crone, enchantress and mothers. Alongside are yantra drawings of the geometric shapes of the yoga goddesses. There are dried fruits and dark chocolate in wooden bowls. Yoga mats are laid out in a circle around the centrepiece with blankets, bolsters and meditation stools.

Half an hour before the start, as invited, people begin to arrive. Everyone who has chosen to attend is a woman on her menopause journey. I welcome them and chat to each about their journey here. I am joined by my co-circle holder, so we are calm in the knowledge that we are supporting each other as we hold space for others.

We have time and space for everyone to arrive in good time and settle. The business of travelling across London to get here fades away and I invite the group, including my co-circle holder, to lie down. We have arrived. Now is the time for settling. I invite the group to notice their breathing, the coolness of the air entering and the warmth of the air leaving. To gently acknowledge their bodies as they lie in the room, maybe the coolness on their face or whether they can feel the material of their clothing against their bodies. I then invite them to bring their attention to their hearts.

With their attention settled there, I open one of my favourite poetry books. The invitation is there to listen or not as I share words that connect to the theme of our day together. On completion of the poem I invite the group to bring themselves slowly up to a comfortable seated position, using whichever of the props provided help to bring them into a place of comfort.

I invite them to orient themselves in the room. To notice the open space outside with the birds cheeping, the space inside the room that has been laid out in honour of their presence, and to look around the room at each person who has chosen to have this time together.

It is time for the circle to begin...

It is our wish that in joining us you will experience more of the joys of sitting in circle, both as a participant and as a facilitator. Through reading this book and working through the exercises, we would love for you to be infused with the will and confidence to go out and create circles of your own or deepen your holding capacity.

Now that you have taken your seat in our circle, we will begin.

● EXERCISE: REFLECTION ON THE MAGIC OF CIRCLES

Allow yourself 20 minutes for this exercise. Have a notepad and some pens to hand. If you like to draw, have a variety of different-coloured pens to use for illustration.

Once you have read these words, close your eyes and give yourself space and time to sit with them. When you feel ready, begin to write or draw until you have written everything that you wish to.

Has there ever been a time when you have sat with others and been given space to speak without interruption? A space where nobody gave you advice or suggestions after you spoke? (This does not have to be a specific circle space.) How did it make you feel?

● EXERCISE: SPONTANEOUS CIRCLE TIME

Sometimes circles happen spontaneously at a social gathering. Imagine this situation.

We are sitting around a dinner table. The first course, soup, has been eaten. Those gathered are from different generations. There are grandparents, parents and teenagers present from different families with some extended family members and friends present without their parents or children. There are about 15 people present. Knowing that there are some people in the gathering who are less familiar with the group and to foster connection, the host quietens the room and asks:

'I would love to go round the table and hear about your connection to me and anyone else sitting around this table.'

Each person speaks, and through their talking connections are made and stories told and listened to that enhance the experience of being together. Rather than only hearing from and speaking to the person on either side of us, we have the experience of all being together as a micro community. Every generation of person present is listened to with the same attentiveness.

Can you remember a time when you experienced circle time, however informal or spontaneous?

Over the next couple of weeks try this exercise with others. If there are a few of you who are looking to create a circle together, find a suitable time and space to gather. A space where you can easily listen to each other. While writing this book, we have both had informal conversations with friends and family about the experience of being in circle: circle time is often filled with stories from our lives. This chapter has shown the magic of being in circle time and that circles can be spontaneous and simple.

Now let's turn to when we create talking and listening circles with intention. In the next chapter we will look at your intention for running a circle and making a start.

CHAPTER 3

Intention Setting – Why Do You Want to Facilitate a Circle?

Perhaps you find yourself in this situation: you're interested in facilitating a talking circle and yet so many questions arise that you feel blocked from taking the next step. Maybe you've fallen into leading circles and want to clarify how circle holding fits into your work and life. In this chapter, we focus on the power of intention and finding your purpose.

In our training courses about circle facilitation, the answer to so many questions comes from having clarity about your intention for the circle. These questions include:

- How do I create a theme for my circle?

- How long should the circle run for?

- How do I communicate that this event exists?

- How do I find people to come to the circle?

- How much should I charge, or should it be free?

It might be tempting to skip ahead to reading about how to open the gathering by establishing the circle guidelines or how to navigate the dynamics of the participants. However, the time that you spend reflecting on the purpose of your circle will be repaid many times over.

● EXERCISE: CONNECTING WITH YOUR PURPOSE

You will need 30 minutes in a quiet space, a notepad and pen, and you may wish to have a large piece of paper with colouring pens.

There are two ways to approach this exercise. You can use either or both.

Intuitive approach

Read this exercise through and then take a moment to close your eyes and dream. Sit in a comfortable position somewhere you can look out into the middle distance.

Allow your focus to come to your breathing. Maybe notice the air as it flows in through your nose and the quality of that air. It might be possible to experience the coolness as it flows into your nostrils. Notice the air as it leaves.

Now allow yourself to imagine the circle you would like to create. Who is sitting with you? Is it a large group or small? What are the points of connection between people? Are you part of the demographic or not? Notice how you feel amongst these people. What has brought you here?

What do you long to share with these people? What does your heart call you to say to them? If you were welcoming them into this circle for the first time, how might you thank them for their presence? Can you imagine the place where you are gathering?

Take your time.

Now write down what came up in a stream of consciousness without editing or judging.

In a moment you'll close your eyes again and focus on WHY you want to hold this circle. What is the underlying reason that you feel called to do this? What need does it fulfil in you?

Write down your reflections. Now put that writing away and give yourself a day away from the words before coming back to them and seeing what gifts they have brought you.

Step-by-step approach

Take a few minutes to write detailed responses to each of these questions. You can always come back and add to your responses later as your ideas take shape.

Who is the circle for? (Try to be specific – either a certain demographic, like new parents, teens or people who have experienced divorce, or people with a specific interest.)

Why do you want to hold a circle? (What is the underlying need that facilitating a circle will fulfil for you and for those participating?)

What is the circle for? What need will it meet in you and what need would you like it to meet in others who attend? (Is there a shared interest that brings you together?)

Keep your thoughts on this in a safe place as this creates the foundations on which you will build your circle.

It is likely that you will be creating your circle out of a personal need, wish or desire.

CIRCLE STORY: HOW TESSA'S RED TENT CAME ABOUT
Tessa shares:

> I started my Red Tent out of a personal need to connect with other women in my community of different ages and out of a wish to learn more about others' experience of menstrual cycle awareness. I started the puberty circles with tweens because of a desire to provide girls with the knowledge that I saw was so valuable to women in the Red Tent.

> I began charting my menstrual cycle with a view to conceiving. Two babies later, I came across *Yoni Shakti* by Uma Dinsmore-Tuli and read about a wider focus on menstrual cycle awareness than fertility alone. I also read the novel *The Red Tent* by Anita Diamont and loved the idea of having regular female company after moving to a new town.

> At the time, the nearest Red Tent circle to me was in St Albans, which was too far away to attend with little children needing me. I decided to take the plunge and start my own. Although I had attended circles as part of workshops and retreats as a participant, I hadn't seen any workshops on how to facilitate one. I hoped that my experience of holding space as a yoga teacher would support me.

> At first I invited friends, neighbours and people in my yoga class to attend. I held it in one of the venues I taught yoga in, pushing the

sofas together and bringing red, pink and purple cushions and fabrics to transform the atmosphere of the place. The lights could be turned down. However, after a couple of sessions, I decided it wasn't cosy enough and the circle stayed in my living room for over a year.

As the numbers grew, we moved to a yurt on the edge of a wood. With a wood stove, this created a special atmosphere and we stayed there until the first lockdown. Then it went online through the pandemic and nine years later (in 2023) is still going strong. I no longer call it a Red Tent, but we still often use the menstrual or lunar cycle as a way of orienting ourselves at the beginning of the cycle. My intention to learn about my menstrual cycle through others' experiences is still there, particularly as it shifts into perimenopause.

When a question arises in the women's circle that can't be answered by the experience of those present, Tessa may share some relevant information. However, her teaching happens in separate workshops because the circle space is for shared experience rather than for one person to dominate. However, it may be that you want to introduce circle time into a workshop, training or retreat to have space to share experiences around the content, and that's fine too.

If you are already a teacher of yoga, tai chi, meditation or something else, your teaching can grow through feedback from students in a circle format. Encouraging sharing around the experience of movement, meditation and deep relaxation can deepen the students' practice also. Julia says:

I remember a time when I decided to deepen my knowledge of meditation. The first evening I attended we were sitting in a circle of chairs. We would take part in a different meditation practice each week and after each practice we would go round the circle and share our experience. My positive experience encouraged me to teach in that way.

Finding your purpose

When you are inviting people to your circle, they will need to understand its purpose so they can decide whether it is right for them. The clearer you are about your purpose, the more likely you are to have people who share that purpose attend and for your circle to succeed.

You might be looking for a place of belonging where experiences can be shared. Throughout this book we share examples of circles that have been created out of a specific need. All of the circle holders have either seen a need in themselves or in others that was met through the creation of circle:

> The intention of the circle was to bring our core humanity, our vulnerability, the truth of our story into the space and it blew me away because of its simplicity.
>
> *Gemma Brady, founder of Sister Stories*

> I have used circle work as a midwife particularly working around the world with different communities talking about certain subjects that are sensitive and in need of a diverse listening to.
>
> *Israh Goodall*

> I do feel boys are in such need of circle time. My experience has been that when held well they deeply appreciate this space.
>
> *Israh Goodall*

> It was in the early 80s. Someone said to me, 'Would you like to be in a circle about feminine spirituality?'
>
> *Suzan Nolan*

> The one place that I participate in my community is a group of men and women who have a common focus which I think is a really important piece of a circle...the focus is the advancement of the community, for it to be inclusive of everyone to move the community forward.
>
> *Mary Thorp*

Here are some examples of talking circles that come from some of the people interviewed in the making of this book and from our own experience. You might see one of these and feel in your heart that this is the circle of belonging you would like to create, or maybe there is another purpose that sings to you. The need that is often met in these circles is to share common experiences.

- Bereavement (grief) circle.

- Breathwork circle – sharing experiences of breathwork practices.

- Celebration Day for Girls – for tweens to learn about puberty and periods.

- Cycle circle – to talk about the experience of having a menstrual cycle.

- Dual heritage circle.

- Embodiment circle – for people who are part of a community of like-minded people looking for body–mind connection.

- Grandmothers' circle – for female elders in their respective communities.

- Groves – for those who support the TreeSisters charity.

- LGBTQIA+ adult community circle – fulfilling the need for the LGBTQIA+ community to meet in settings outside of the clubbing scene.

- Menarche circle – for pre-teens and their parents.

- Menopause circle – for those experiencing perimenopause and menopause.

- Multigenerational circles – with a specific focus for their community, such as the needs of their teenage boys.

- New moon or menstruality circle or Red Tent – themes around menstruation.

- New parents circle – with yoga and baby massage, but mainly to talk.

- Parent circle – for parents with pre-school children interested in attachment parenting.

- Positive sexuality circle – for practising language around consent and touch.

- Pregnancy circle – to explore the experience of being pregnant and previous birthings.

- Story circles – to explore experience through listening to stories.

- Teen boys coming-of-age circles.

- Women's circle – for women to gather and share authentically from the heart.

All of these examples are represented through stories and quotations throughout this book. Many facilitators created their circle from a specific personal need. For example, Daniel Groom, co-founder of Queer Wellbeing, said, 'I set it up because it is what I needed. Circle holding is a gateway to other ways for the community to come together. Creating a space for people to have a voice. Creating options outside of nightclubs.'

Tanya Forgan created the community Blended Roots to run circles for women of dual/mixed heritage. This came out of her need for a way in which to address difficult conversations around race and belonging, conversations that have proven to be healing and helpful: 'The absence of spaces catering for me stemmed from the fact that the circles I frequented mainly consisted of white women. Consequently, it didn't feel safe for me to openly share any experiences regarding race or racism.'

Sometimes the challenge experienced in a circle space leads to an intention to meet a need that is not being met.

When we interviewed circle holders, some remembered beautiful experiences of being in circle that they wanted to emulate, and others went back to times when they felt unheard and unseen. Mark Walsh of Embodiment Unlimited said:

> A lot of my whole life's work is a reaction to my education experience in a state school – stiff, controlling, bullied by teachers... One or two teachers held discussions instead. It felt freer and more respectful. The first inkling that something else was possible.

The more positive experiences of talking circles that we hear about, the more we may feel emboldened in this work, coming together to make a difference to the lives of those who attend and the ripple effect of that. A participant in an international women's circle said:

> It [being in circle] helps me stay grounded. I notice a very subtle shifting within me. I am becoming a better listener. I am not giving as much advice. I am becoming clearer about my own purpose...the residual effect of circle is magical to me... The sweetness of life is showing itself to me... I believe deep in my heart that it is a result of attending circles.

Another participant said:

> Sitting in circle is the space that is changing the world... We are holding space for all these people and these issues in our world and I feel like I have this knowing inside that the more that we sit in circle the more chance we have to save our world.

Sometimes an intention for a circle will be grand in scale. For example, the TreeSisters charity aims to reforest the tropics to support the environment globally. Their circles are called Groves and support the inner work of the people who donate to the cause.

Other times, the intention for a circle will be for a small number of people to come together. The 'No Club' was created by five professional women who found themselves doing way too many non-promotable tasks in work. Their circle proved so successful in its mission that they helped other women create 'No Clubs' to help women to say no to non-promotable tasks. They created guidelines on the size of the group and its diversity, and advised that the group would be more likely to succeed if kept exclusively female.

With both of these examples, you may have noticed that the intention of the circles was very specific and the nature of their intention had a significant impact on the kind of circle created.

Reflect about why you want to hold a circle. Be specific about your intention and look at ways of framing that purpose for others. You can create your circle and bring in those people for whom it will serve. Here's a final example of someone who didn't set out to lead a circle at all.

CIRCLE STORY: CYCLE CIRCLE AT SCHOOL

Anouska is 17 years old and a couple of years ago one of her teachers began a small group called the Cycle Circle. Of all the clubs in school, she told me that this one is not advertised. Students at her all-girls school find out about the circle by word of mouth. There is no cost to attend and it takes place every Tuesday lunchtime.

She described how the circle is facilitated by her teacher and they physically sit in a circle. Each girl is invited to share the day they are in their menstrual cycle (with day 1 being the first day of their bleed) and how they feel, using the seasons as a reference. The seasons are explained in terms of the menstrual cycle: spring (pre-ovulation), summer (ovulation), autumn (pre-menstruum), and winter (bleed time).

Through being part of this circle she has gained a deeper understanding of her body and her hormones, and particularly how her mood is affected by the ebb and flow of her cycle. She has now become a leader in menstrual education within her school. This has involved giving talks to the girls in Year 7 and Year 8 (age 11–13) about periods. Her school funded the purchase of a wide variety of menstrual products, including menstrual cups and period pants, so that the older girls could educate the girls further down the school. The teacher is now wondering how the older girls can facilitate circles for the younger students.

Anouska realised that the skills she gained as a youth movement leader within her religious community lent themselves beautifully to running circles of her own; she just hadn't thought of it like that before. Her experience of being held in circle and holding circles of her own as a teenager stands her in good stead for later positive leadership roles.

⬤ EXERCISE: INTENTION SETTING

Now that you've read about other circle holders' intentions for setting up a diverse range of gatherings, take some time to become very clear on your intention. Here are some questions to help you:

- What are your reasons for wanting to facilitate a circle? (Does it fulfil a need for yourself and/or serve others in some way?)

- Has reading through the examples of different intentions for circles changed your intention? If so, how?

- How specific can you make your intention?

- Can you word your most important reason for facilitating a circle as an affirmation? (e.g. 'I need a space to be with other dual heritage women where I feel safe' could become 'As a dual heritage woman, I create a safe space to share experiences of race and belonging'.)

It can be helpful to look at your intention in terms of aims and objectives. For example:

Aim: To create a space where new parents can share their experience to support each other in their wish to practise attachment parenting.

Objective: By the end of the circle we will have spoken about a specific aspect of attachment parenting and addressed challenges we are facing.

Now see whether you can turn your intention into an aim and an objective. Don't worry about it being perfect. This exercise is for your own clarification and not to share with anyone else.

Once we have become clear about what we would like to happen, we can begin to create an environment where the aim or dream can become reality.

Inclusivity in circles

Inclusion is the aim to enable access regardless of personal, physical and social characteristics.

Your original intention for holding a circle is important here. A circle may be open to anyone and everyone or it may be aimed at a specific demographic such as new parents, people who identify as LGBTQIA+, those grieving or those with a specific interest such as menstrual cycle awareness. If you are clear on your intention, then it is easier to consider within those parameters how you can be as inclusive as possible. Daniel Groom says, 'Pronouns at the start of a circle can be an affirming and inclusive way to make LGBTQIA+ people feel welcome.'

Inclusion can be confusing because the main narrative we hear is that everything should be accessible to everyone all the time. This can make calling something a 'men's circle' or 'women's circle' seem wrong. It is okay to have a certain demographic in mind.

It is common for groups that serve a very specific demographic to be led by people who have experience of that characteristic or lived experience. For example, those running a grief circle will have experienced loss. If you are choosing to run a circle for people and you do not have shared experience, you may wish to have the intention to train someone from that demographic in circle facilitation who can take over the role.

> It's important to have facilitators who are trained from the communities too. I am a white middle-aged guy: it's not going to be as easy for me to facilitate a space for kids who grew up in gangs, for example, so why don't we train people up who come from that community and have them lead and model the process.
>
> *Lee Keylock*

Another example is the Happy Baby Community, a charity for refugees. It was initially led by people who were not from the refugee community, and over the years more and more of the people who hold space have experienced the services they provide.

Many organisations also thrive through people coming up through the ranks as it were, from new person to someone with years of experience in that context. This can build a sustainable community, especially if your circle is in the charity sector where you are donating your time and burnout can occur. Even if you are running a small local circle, if you have long-term attendees, they can become co-facilitators and take on the circle if you are unwell or away.

● EXERCISE: INCREASING INCLUSION FOR MY DEMOGRAPHIC

Take time to read through the questions and write down or draw your responses.

- Will your circle welcome people with physical differences? (If so, how will they access the circle and are they able to take part in all activities?)

- Are your activities accessible for all? (e.g. Have you included writing activities which could exclude people with dyslexia?)

- If you are serving a demographic that you do not yourself belong to, do you need to co-facilitate with someone who does?

- If everyone looks the same in your circle, are the images you are using to promote your circle showing diversity? Do you explain who is welcome?

- If you are looking to attract people with differing finances, would a sliding scale for payment help? Is the circle located and advertised in places that are likely to attract a diverse group?

- If your circle is not diverse, would you like any of the proceeds from your group to go to another that serves a more marginalised community?

You might not have answers for all these questions, but hopefully they are thought-provoking and you can return to them as your circle matures. Reaching out to the people you see are not attending can give you ideas about why they don't feel the circle is for them.

We think being clear about your intention for the circle is pivotal in so many decisions you'll make about the circle. Now that you've become clearer about why you want to run the circle and who you want to run it for, in the next chapter we will look at how to overcome common emotional blocks to getting started.

CHAPTER 4

I Want to Run a Circle – Feel the Fear and Go for It!

As you contemplate holding a circle, perhaps there are different, contrasting emotions coming up. You want to be a facilitator and you wonder if you're ready. You hope to bring people together in community and you feel like an imposter. You want everything to be perfect and yet you've never done this before. This is all normal and part of the journey. In this chapter, we explore the feelings around leadership and circle facilitation.

In our workshops, participants often worry about whether they are qualified enough to facilitate a circle. They might be thinking about qualification in terms of having the right piece of paper to show others evidence of their capacity or skill. Or perhaps meaning it in a broader sense: do they know enough to do a good job? As far as we're aware, there is no country that has an accrediting or governing body for circle holding, and if they did, that might have prevented some of those people who have shared their stories with us from starting. Those for whom circle formed an integral part of their formative years felt a natural progression towards running circle themselves, but even they felt nerves when they stepped into the role of facilitator.

Increasingly, there are training courses to support people in feeling confident to hold different types of circles. Some may seek accreditation from the awarding bodies for other disciplines, such as Mandy Ree's Mother Circle, which is certified by the International Association of Therapists. However, there is not a national organisation that sets standards to be attained and neither should there be. Often organisations that run circles require the circle holder to have trained in a specific skill set, and often they will need to be part of the demographic they serve. This is true in the case of Alcoholics Anonymous and Support after Murder and Manslaughter.

If a specific training is not required, you might feel unqualified and subconsciously hold off the moment of facilitating the circle. Our aim is to help you feel brave enough to try. It does not need to be in any way perfect. You will make mistakes. You will have building blocks of holding a circle and see the mistakes others have made and learn from them. Let's look at the common feelings that come up.

Nervousness

Stepping into a circle as a facilitator for the first time can feel like stepping on to a stage for the first night of a play or having to stand in front of a group to give a presentation. You have sent an invitation out to others, and your biggest fear may not actually be that nobody comes but the opposite: for the room to be full of people with expectation. At that very moment of the circle beginning, your heart might be in your mouth.

Gemma Brady of Sister Stories shares how she felt when she ran her first circle: 'Like I was standing on the precipice of holding something, like that, thinking this could go in any direction. I have no control. As a first-time facilitator it was terrifying.'

She further remembers:

It is not appealing to me to be in a room where I share my voice and people listen. It is not the way I am inclined at all and so I can remember my voice shaking when I opened the space.

And the way that I handled that was to acknowledge and name it: 'It is hard for me to share my voice, maybe it is hard for you to do that too. This is a space where we can allow them to wobble, where we can feel nervous, where we allow ourselves to experiment with opening our mouths and see what comes out.'

And from day one in that circle, it felt really important to me: not pretending to be anything other than I was.

Some of the people we interviewed would describe themselves as introverts, highly sensitive people and empaths; others are natural extroverts. We are drawn to communicating in meaningful ways, taking in the non-verbal information and dynamics, and enjoy listening and learning from others. Having the structure of a circle, which we'll unpick in later chapters, can help to keep a group situation from becoming overwhelming, not only for facilitators but, more importantly, for all involved. In part, this is because people don't talk over each other and interrupt.

For Israh Goodall, the transformative moment was being asked, as a 26-year-old, to hold a circle for a community in Switzerland. She says:

> I remember being invited to hold a women's circle by some of the elders of that community and it was so extraordinarily terrifying, AND I knew that it was the right moment and the right situation. Every part of my body was on fire. I could feel something deep in me was being rattled.
>
> That was the first time I had held a group with women of all ages and backgrounds from all around the world, sitting in circle in the mountains. I remember really landing in my destiny. The sense of okay. This is part of the way I am going to move in the world.

She felt nervous and did it anyway.

Acknowledging the possibility of people being nervous could help you as you approach your circle holding. A common thread amongst participants in listening circles is that the first time it can feel vulnerable, uncomfortable and even a little unsafe. An experience that is new can bring about these feelings in facilitators too:

> I don't have experience of circle holding so I'm quite nervous about it, especially in terms of timing and making sure people feel listened to and heard but not allowing for people to talk for too long. Also I'm unsure about how to hold space for any big things that might come up or for a lot of emotions. One of my biggest challenges would be getting people's interest and establishing myself as someone who offers/runs circles.

Frankie Culpin

> The thought of a sharing circle was very intimidating until I was part of one. My biggest concerns are making people feel uncomfortable and under pressure to share and also someone sharing something so enormous or traumatic that I don't know what to do with it.

Anonymous

Another tip is to prepare the participants before they attend circle. When you speak to people about your gathering in advance, you could ask them what piqued their interest. This would also give you an opportunity to introduce yourself and hear about them so that you won't be sitting in circle time with a group of complete strangers. We will talk later about marketing and outlining expectations for a gathering.

If the gathering is online and time-limited, with people invited along for a specific number of weeks or months, you might invite people into a WhatsApp group or online closed space where they can all share a photo of themselves and their reasons for joining the circle before the first one begins. This will give them a sense of the community they have joined and will give you a clearer idea of who will belong to your circle. The clearer the expectations at the start, the more comfortable all will be about the gathering itself, including you.

1. Set expectations in your invitation.

2. Have clear guidelines you explain at the beginning of your circle.

3. Think about whether you would like a little informal time before the circle begins to allow for a settling of nerves.

4. Set the scene and give yourself and your nervous system time to settle at the beginning of each circle.

The fewer unknowns there are about the structure and theme, the more comfortable those attending will be. We will be unpacking this over the coming chapters.

If you choose to speak to someone on the phone before a circle, it's important to set boundaries for the communication. For example, if you say that you would like to find out about each other over a brief telephone call, say specifically that it will take ten minutes maximum and stick to it.

Addressing the deep fear of circle holding

For some of the people we interviewed, the fear of facilitating went beyond the anxiety around public speaking and being the focus of attention. A deeper-rooted fear was named: the past persecution of wise women. The special space that can be created through listening circles can be reminiscent of those held by herbalists, midwives and other powerful women in the community that religion feared.

> I live in an ultra-conservative area, and when I started doing circles, I was very secretive about this and I did not feel safe. You know, from the burning times. Women's spirituality, women sitting in circle. We have

been cast as witches, as evil, hags and much worse. They were certainly suspicious of the mischief we might be doing in these circles.

Suzan Nolan

I had this fear of persecution for holding this kind of space. The 'Witch Wound' feeling.

Gemma Brady

One way of addressing this deep fear is to seek out others who hold circles and avoid being isolated. The fear may be compounded by other layers of persecution, such as being from a minority group who are often denied a voice.

Fear often has a root of truth. There may be circles that you would like to run that you are not quite ready for.

Before Julia began to run circles around the menstrual cycle, she took time to unpack her personal experience of being put on the pill at 14, issues around conception, chronic illness and her own daughter's experience of menarche (first bleed). It was at this stage that she felt ready to run circles on this topic.

Tessa felt ready to run kids' circles once her children were of an age to attend them because she understood more clearly how to respond to their needs and deliver age-appropriate content, and had found a love for the craft activities that worked well with this demographic.

Do you need to be an expert?

Yes and no!

It all depends on the purpose of your circle.

However, there are many circumstances in which expertise in the subject of circle is not required, but forming part of the demographic for that circle is. For example, if you are not part of the LGBTQIA+ community, it is unlikely you would set up a circle for that community. If you do not menstruate, you are unlikely to set up a menstruality circle. Not only would it be unlikely for you to make that choice, but you would also be very unlikely to attract people to your intended circle.

It is a different experience running a circle and holding a space for others (e.g. a pregnancy circle when you are not pregnant), and holding a circle of your peers. In the former, you have likely been in that position in the past, but not necessarily. In the latter, you will be contributing and taking part in circle as a participant as well as the founder of the group. Having lived experience of the topic being brought to the circle may give you credibility as a facilitator, although it could also free you to not have current or past lived experience, but curiosity. There is no one right answer.

> I am not in perimenopause, I am in a different space – it is no longer that I am going to speak in that way. I share how I am feeling – I share what is going on with me within the circle. I don't share my lived experience.
>
> *Kate Codrington*

The intention is to create egalitarian spaces where everyone can be equally heard. There might be situations where you combine teaching with circle time. In this case, you would have expertise about what you are teaching, but be aware of the dynamic that this sets up in the circle space. It may be that the presence of your 'expertise' potentially shuts down others' voices; we will share techniques you can use to help prevent this from happening.

If the circle has been created as a learning tool for others, then there will be an expectation and need for expertise. Julia uses circle time as part of her Perimenopause Yoga Facilitator training, and there is an expectation amongst participants that they will learn specific knowledge and skills they can use with their own community. The marketing for the training is specific and clear about the knowledge that will be shared.

Guidelines are shared at the start of the training and live participation is required. From the first session, the intention is for all of those taking part to notice how beneficial it is to hear the voices of everyone who has joined the training, and that will bring a richness to the learning that the content alone cannot provide. However, without the expertise of the trainers, the aims and objectives of the training would not be fulfilled.

Whether people pay or not also comes into play here. (The issue of charging will be discussed in detail in Chapter 18.) If you charge for the circle, there may be more expectation of responsibility and of greater skill than for a free gathering.

It is okay to be transparent and share that you are new to circle facilitation. Sharing your nervousness can break down the feeling of 'you' and 'them', or 'the expert' and 'the others', and support sharing.

Go for it! Preventing procrastination

Part of the block around expertise may be due to a trait of perfectionism. If you are someone that wants everything to look professional, flow seamlessly and seem as if you have been doing it for years, please accept that you are in a learning phase.

In one of Tessa's workshops on circle holding, Csilla, who runs girls' circles and mother circles, shared that she was struggling with wanting everything to be perfect before she started. She wanted to know how to get everything in the right order during the circle and know what activities and topics would work for her groups. Tessa responded, 'Trial and error. You know by testing it out and asking for feedback.' This was a lightbulb moment for Csilla and gave her tremendous permission to not get it right from the beginning.

It's also common to experience imposter syndrome when starting to lead circles. You may feel that by guiding the gathering you are expressing a state of wisdom that you don't actually feel. Being open about your feelings, as Gemma Brady did above, can set the scene for authentic communication.

CIRCLE STORY: START BEFORE YOU ARE READY

Julia once hosted a Moon Circle where the theme was 'Start Before You Are Ready'. She had become aware of her fear of doing things because of an innate feeling that she lacked the qualifications. She wanted to regain some of the fearlessness she had as a teenager and young woman – a time in life when many of us feel fearless because our prefrontal cortex is not yet fully developed and we are naturally seeking dopamine. (The 'happy hormone' dopamine is the primary driver of the brain's reward system.)

In the Moon Circle, participants looked at what held them back and drew and painted self-portraits. There were a wide variety of pictures created. Bravery was required to put pen to paper. None of us were artists! Once the pictures were drawn, we talked about how it felt to create the picture. By the end of the circle, the fears associated with feeling under-qualified to take a step were addressed and it was recognised that sometimes what is needed is bravery rather than qualifications. Attendees were then invited to remember their favourite teachers: those who not only knew their subject but who listened to you, had fun and fostered community. Those skills are needed far more than perfectionism or getting things just right.

We tend to be very forgiving of people who do something from their heart, and that is exactly what we are aiming to foster in talking circles: listening skills and speaking from the heart.

EXERCISE: YOUR EXPERIENCE OF BEING HELD

Read through these instructions and then close your eyes or look into the middle distance. Take a breath and find a comfortable position to settle in.

See whether you can take your mind back to a time when you had the experience of being emotionally held. This may not be in a listening circle space or group situation. It may be a one-to-one encounter. If you can remember a time like this, sense how it felt in your body. If you can't, you could read the descriptions of the magic of being in circle in Chapter 2 and imagine or think about what that would be like. Be as specific as you can about how it feels to be in this space and what contributes to making that possible. Write down in a stream of consciousness or draw pictures (without editing or judgement).

Now shift to remembering a time when you created that space to be emotionally held for someone else or a group of people. Again, it does not need to be in a circle setting. What qualities did you draw on? Do any of these words resonate: patient, compassionate, spacious, grounded, centred, calm, mindful, fun, exciting, moving, beautiful? How does this feel in your body? Write down in a stream of consciousness what came up or draw pictures.

CIRCLE STORY: TESSA'S FIRST CIRCLE EXPERIENCE

I was always shy as a child. As a 16-year-old, I took my work experience at an architect's practice and would make the manager jump every time I went into his office. I would silently walk up to the desk for fear of interrupting and then he'd leap out of his seat when he glanced up. My teachers are unlikely to have imagined I would become a circle holder and leader!

I don't remember exactly the very first time I was in a talking circle – it would have been at one of the women's retreats I went on during my thirties. The first circle I do clearly remember was part of a training around menstrual cycle awareness, and there were more than 20 women in the room, with two facilitating. I remember the end of one day when we'd been diving deep into our experiences of the menstrual cycle and big emotions were coming up. We were doing a final circle before finishing for dinner, sharing how we were feeling and what we'd learnt from the day.

In the past, I would have felt a mounting pressure to say the right thing so I wouldn't be judged as being out of place. This time I felt a deep acceptance of myself and that it was okay not to know what to say, not to saying anything if I didn't want to and that the others could take or leave what I said.

I didn't spend the time thinking about what I was going to say when it was my turn, but really listened to the others. When it was my turn, I paused, sensing into what it was exactly I was feeling. It wasn't particularly profound, but it was my truth at that moment in time. It was wonderful to feel authentically me.

This experience was enabled partly by the skilled facilitators and partly through the journey I'd been on through multiple circles to accept that I am okay as I am. To anyone listening in that circle, it wouldn't have seemed like a pivotal moment, but it's after this that I decided to run my own circle. I was ready.

Hopefully, by sharing my journey, you can see that being ready to facilitate is part of a process often without a clear beginning and end.

Receiving a certificate is a moment in time. Without diminishing the helpfulness of training, developing the qualities for circle holding is ongoing and mostly experiential. Taking that first step has proven so transformative for many circle holders in this book. We have your back: we have been there and understand the bravery that may be needed.

● EXERCISE: REFLECTIONS ON FEELING THE FEAR AND DOING IT ANYWAY

Give yourself 15 minutes of uninterrupted time. Take a notepad and pen or large sheet and colouring pens and write your responses to the questions or draw pictures to illustrate them.

- ● What blocks have you identified to starting your circle or taking your work to the next level?

- What positive experiences can you draw on to give you confidence, whether they're in a circle setting or in a different group scenario?

- Who can inspire you as a circle facilitator or leader?

- How have the stories in the book so far shown you that being a circle holder is a journey rather than a destination?

EXERCISE: REMOVING OBSTACLES AND MOVING FORWARD

You might want to do this exercise with friends, other circle holders or circle participants. It is a wonderful activity to create a feeling of transformation.

Ask people to write down everything that is blocking them and around a particular issue. Try to be as specific as possible about the obstacles.

Now invite your participants to start with one specific obstacle and write an action to overcome it. Make it a small, achievable step with a time frame. If you have time, create more actions. Come back to the circle and share your action plan.

If you have the right venue for this, the obstacles can be written on paper and set alight by a candle or in a fire pit and burnt. The facilitator can write one word about an individual's action on a piece of coloured card and create a centrepiece of all the people's intentions.

When we have blocks, finding ways to take action can be a really useful way to address those blocks.

EXERCISE: EMBODIED SUPPORT

This is a practice you can do in a group of three or more. Stand in your group and each of you can stand on one leg and see how long you can balance for. You can do this in any way – you might like to use the tree pose that is commonly used in yoga practice. When you do this, it is helpful to look at a spot in the middle distance to help you balance.

Now come into a circle. Each of you decide which leg you will stand on and come into your balance. Now place your left hand and touch it to the right hand of the person next to you – so that each person has their left hand flat against the next person's right. See how long you can balance in the circle.

If people can balance quite easily, you can put in intentional movement. Imagine trees blowing in the wind. You could see how well the forest can be sustained with movement too!

What happens when you balance in this way is that you support each other and in this way are able to stay in the circle far longer. This can be sustained with small and large numbers of people. It reminds us that when we do things alone we can only last for so long. With support of our community, we can both give and receive, allowing us to be sustained for a longer period.

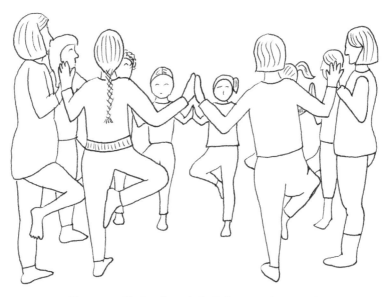

Figure 4.1 Circle of people in Vrksasana (tree pose)

You may have noticed, now that we are at Chapter 4, all the exercises we share here can be practised in a talking circle, and it might be fun to bring friends together who are also interested in circle holding to compare your answers.

This chapter acknowledges the challenging feelings that may arise when you contemplate being a facilitator responsible for holding space and encourages you to go ahead anyway. Facilitation doesn't happen in a vacuum, and if you're holding regular circles, it's normal to feel that some were held more effectively than others.

Lee Keylock has been involved in Narrative 4 for ten years. Narrative 4 is a non-profit organisation that builds a culture of connection through the power of storytelling. It offers a wide array of programmes which help develop the essential practices of deep listening, curiosity, imagination and positive action (see narrative4.com). Lee says this about his sessions:

> We don't have a magic wand. We are not perfect at it either. Did all the facilitations look pretty? No, of course not. I screwed up so many times that I can't even tell you. But you learn. We put more infrastructure in place. More safeguards and parameters around things.

The more you understand the different components that can create the container of a circle, the more structure you are creating to support your facilitation. We will take you through the process of opening your circle, sharing guidelines, introducing the talking and listening, and closing. We start in Chapter 5 with exploring how to set up your circle.

Setting Up for Your Circle

The space is quiet and ordinary. There is a temptation to rush in and organise the seating, get the kettle on, set up this and that, but pausing allows the intentions for the circle to be remembered. With slow breaths and checking in with your body you find there are different emotions present: maybe anticipation, nervousness, hopefulness... Then into action to create a welcoming space for those who have taken this brave step of joining a talking circle.

Unless you are running a collaborative circle where everyone is involved in helping to set up the space, time for you to prepare the venue and create the right atmosphere before everyone arrives is important.

How to physically arrange a circle

By its nature, a listening circle happens in a physical circle so that all can be seen and heard.

In Elif Shafak's book *Three Daughters of Eve* (2016) a tutor gets everyone to rearrange their chairs: 'But God had to be discussed in a circle, everyone on the circumference equidistant from the centre, looking at one another's eyes' (p. 221).

Whatever is being discussed, being in a circular shape makes a big difference, so change the room layout if necessary. Sitting around regular tables will make people think of school and work meetings and change the dynamics.

Depending on who is coming to the circle, it may be appropriate to sit in chairs or to sit on the floor with various props. There may be a low table for a centrepiece, but usually bigger tables will be avoided because they create a barrier between people.

Setting up the room beforehand for the number of participants who will be there is helpful so that there are no gaps between seats and the participants are spaced evenly. If anyone is absent when the circle begins the empty chair can be removed. We strongly recommend that you visit the venue before the event. Check the acoustics in the room so that it is as easy as possible for the participants to hear each other and notice if there are any external sounds that could interfere. More on this in Chapter 18 on logistics.

Check that chairs are comfortable for an extended time. In someone's home or some venues, a variety of different seated options may be available. If you're planning to sit on the floor, make sure that enough cushions, bolsters and meditation stools/floor chairs are available and consider what alternative there could be for someone with less mobility. Julia has a variety of blankets, blocks, meditation stools and bolsters in her studio to enable comfort when sitting. Chairs are very rarely used in her studio but can be used when all other forms of sitting do not bring the required comfort.

You can ask people to bring cushions with them: when Tessa ran her women's circle in a yurt on the edge of a wood, the women would bring whatever they needed to make themselves comfortable. There were a few uncomfortable chairs in there, but we preferred to sit on the floor with some using meditation chairs and most using a couple of cushions and a blanket for cosiness.

Tanya Forgan remembers:

> One evening there were fewer people [at the mindfulness training] and I said, 'Let's put the chairs together and sit in a circle.' I remember then, I had a visceral feeling that something had changed in this space. It was transformative for how I took things forward.

It is possible to run circles that are part in person and part online. In this case, a semi-circle of chairs facing a large screen where you can see the online participants could work (see Chapter 16 on online circles for more guidance). In the case of mixing in person and online, it is important that those attending online can hear the people in the room. This is a specific challenge that occurs when mixing online and in person, and you may need to buy a good-quality microphone for this purpose.

For circles where babies and children are welcome, creating a space for them to feel comfortable (e.g. with age-appropriate toys or activities, changing facilities) and where parents can comfortably feed is wonderful. Some circles provide a creche for children to one side of the room so parents can focus on being part of a gathering for themselves (see the circle story 'Becoming mums and the mothers' quilt' in Chapter 13).

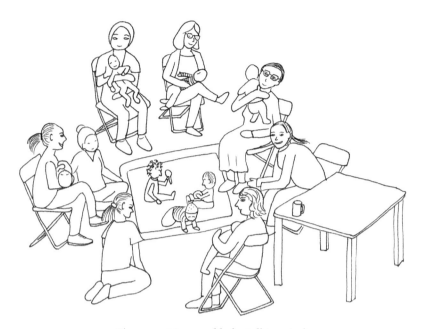

Figure 5.1 Mum and baby talking circle

It might be that part of your talking circle involves making things. In this case, you might need tables to work on. You may want to factor in additional space to accommodate everything. When Tessa runs Celebration Day for Girls, a lot of activity happens in the middle of the circle, with co-creating a mandala, colouring and sharing experiences. However, there's also extra space for dancing and partner yoga to break up the sitting and to gather round to look at period products.

Creating the right atmosphere

It is important that the space you are sharing is clean, clear and tidy, whether you are sharing an in-person or virtual circle. If a venue is used for an everyday purpose, it is helpful to signal that something different is about to happen. For example, one of Tessa's circle holder trainees was a lecturer at a university and created a talking circle for overseas PhD students. They needed to meet in a room that was commonly used for meetings and so she brought some flowers and a cloth for the floor to signal that a different kind of gathering was about to happen.

When Julia shares online circles, she uses throws and pretty blankets to cover any technology in the room and closes the curtains so that her room looks cosy and comfortable. Sometimes it is not possible to be in a place with a background that looks pleasant, so technology can be used to create a background that is conducive to the circle being held.

There are different ways you could change the space into something less functional and more special, or even sacred. Beyond moving the seating into a circle, think about transforming how the space looks, smells and sounds. For changing the look of the room, this might be draping soft materials (also to change the acoustics), bringing cushions and blankets to give a sense of comfort, changing the lighting and bringing relevant objects. Candlelight can be a very special way to create atmosphere.

Creating a centrepiece can give a natural focus to the gathering. Julia has a circular blanket that she often places in the centre of a circle, and items that relate to that week's theme are placed there together with a 'talking stick'. A talking stick or bowl or other object can be picked up by a circle participant when they feel called to speak: this signals that only the person holding the object can speak and the others will listen. Another alternative is to use a card. Julia often brings oracle cards or picture cards into her circle space. She has some beautiful ones depicting the ages of woman and yoga symbols. She often hands them out to participants at the start of the talking circle and someone could lift up their card when they feel moved to speak.

Tessa has found that a talking object hasn't always worked in a circle situation. Especially in a larger circle, it can take time for the object to be passed along, and sometimes this disrupts the flow of talk from one person to another. The talking stick can work well where there is a particular issue to be discussed and it's important to hear everyone's thoughts on it, or where you are hearing each person speak in turn around the circle.

Having the talking object in your hands can give a sense of authority to speak. If you use such an object, make sure you explain the reason for using it at the beginning of the circle. Holding a talking stick can also help prevent interruption: while a person is holding the object, others cannot speak until the object is put down.

A centrepiece could be as simple as a candle or a vase of flowers. You could make a simple display with natural objects such as seasonal flowers, leaves, pebbles, fir cones, acorns, feathers or whatever is to hand. It could also be crystals, oracle cards or objects brought by the attendees relevant to the theme; there are no limits other than your imagination! Having a clean, attractive piece of material will create a good base for whatever you put on top.

In the Hindu and Buddhist traditions, a mandala is a sacred, geometric design often used for meditative practice. It has become used as a word to describe all manner of circular designs, many of which would be suitable as a centrepiece for a talking circle. You can lay out material in the desired shape and then use objects to make symmetrical geometric patterns (see Figure 5.2 for examples of how mandalas looked after co-creation). It is easier if you divide the shape evenly with ribbons or objects to create quarters as a base. You might create the quadrants beforehand and then ask people to take turns creating their own design, replicating it in each of the quarters.

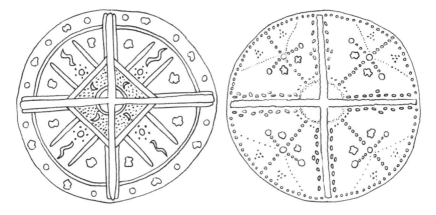

Figure 5.2 Mandalas co-created with rice, beans and lentils in two girls' circles

A fire is a powerful natural centrepiece that brings out something elemental in most people. It can be used as part of the circle process – for example, through burning paper with feelings that people would like to let go of. You might want to ask for a volunteer to look after the fire so that you can concentrate on facilitating.

Participants can be invited to bring flowers, food or objects special to them or related to a theme, but think about how you can set up the space so it already feels welcoming and special for their arrival.

Co-created spaces are wonderful, and requesting support to set up before the official start time and help tidy afterwards is recommended. Everybody could pitch in, or you might offer a discounted place to a helper. Lisa Horwell said, 'The first year I did it on my own. I was doing it on my own and getting resentful.' This can particularly be the case if the circle is run for free or a small donation. While this gift of your time might feel sustainable at the beginning, we invite you to reflect on what will support the longevity of your circle.

Engage the senses

Using the sense of smell can be another way to prepare the space. There are lots of traditions that use scent in sacred gatherings, such as smudge sticks (bundles of sage) used by the Indigenous people of North America to welcome in the four elements, or the herbs frankincense and myrrh in the Catholic Church. Paying tribute to where a tradition has originated is incredibly important, and you may want to discover your own ancestral ways of creating sacred space.

When using incense and oil diffusers, be aware that these might be overpowering or irritating for some people. If you are allowed to use them in a hired venue, we suggest using them before the circle and airing the space, rather than during the gathering itself.

Music can soften people's arrival and create a special atmosphere. Tessa's favourites are the Devi Prayer and Deva Premal's songs. You might choose to share popular music that keeps the energy light. Ensure that you have all the right permissions to play music. You usually need to get a licence if you play recorded music in public or at your business (including background music on a CD, radio or music channel). In the UK, the licence you need is called TheMusicLicence (information from www.gov.uk/licence-to-play-live-or-recorded-music).

Using a sound to mark the start of the circle can create a special atmosphere. You do not need to be a musician to use hand chimes (e.g. bringing them together three times), a singing bowl or hand drum (a low, steady beat to signal the start and stop the chatter). Practising beforehand and having an instrument ready will support your preparations.

It is helpful to create a checklist of what you need to create a welcoming space. You can find one in Chapter 19 where we talk about practical considerations.

● EXERCISE: CANDLE LIGHTING

Many circle holders use candle lighting as a ritual. This can be a beautiful practice to share in an evening circle, and you might not have considered it in the daytime. It can be equally powerful as a practice in the daytime.

The candle is lit to signify the opening of the circle and blown out to denote the end of the circle. When meeting in person, one candle could be used at the centre of the circle. When creating an online gathering, part of the information sent out in preparation for the circle could be to invite people to light their own candle at the start of the gathering.

Take a moment now to find a candle and light it. Notice how this creates a natural pause in what you're doing. It may create a reflective space or make something ordinary like journalling more special.

Tessa likes to place a round mirror horizontally in the centre of the circle and put a bigger 'parent' candle in the middle. A tealight for each attendee is then put around the edge. When doing the initial introductions, each person lights their own tealight from the parent candle. Sometimes, as they do this, they'll be invited to say, 'My name is...and I call myself fully present.' At the end, each person finishes with a few words of how the circle has been and blows their own tealight out.

The yogic practice of candle gazing can be used with one central candle. The gaze goes to the candle wick. This can be used as a settling practice for the group. The participants are invited to gently focus their gaze on the wick of the candle. When they blink, they are invited to keep their eyes closed until whatever image they see behind their closed eyes disappears. They then open their eyes and continue to gaze. The circle holder is responsible for the amount of time the gazing continues for. Two to three minutes can work well. Participants can be invited to share their experience of candle gazing.

The contraindications for candle gazing are cataracts, myopia, glaucoma, astigmatism, epilepsy and wearing contact lenses. Alternatives to candle gazing can be yantra gazing. A yantra is a geometric diagram, usually from the Tantric traditions of yoga and religions of South Asian origin.

When Julia uses candle gazing in circle time, she always has her yantra cards as an alternative practice. The practice of yantra and candle gazing can be a great circle experience. The circle holder talks the participants through the practice and once it is complete, each participant talks about their experience of candle gazing/yantra gazing. They can describe what they saw with their eyes closed, how long the image stayed, what colours they were aware of and how they felt during and after the practice.

Sometimes the colours participants see can be vivid and wonderful and the sense of calm is palpable in the room. Julia has found this practice to be one of the most simple and easy meditation practices for people who are new to a practice that can bring about calm and centring. Sharing the experience of candle or yantra gazing can be an easy gateway to deeper forms of circle sharing – or not. The act of sitting in circle and sharing various focusing, breathing or meditation practices can be the focus of a circle.

Preparing practices such as these and using candles can create a special atmosphere at the beginning of the circle, because humans have always had an important relationship with light and fire.

Preparing yourself for facilitating

Some of us will have been in the situation where we're hosting friends and rushing to get everything done, only to feel frazzled by the time they arrive. An important way of creating a container of safety is for the facilitator to plan time before the circle to settle themselves. This could be ten minutes of becoming still, breathing more slowly and checking in physically and mentally.

Perhaps you have a physical practice like tai chi or yoga, where you could do a couple of movements to bring presence into your body. You may be in a location where you can walk in a garden or a wider open space. Julia likes to walk her dog in the morning before she teaches her classes, in the open air whatever the weather; this grounds her and sets her up.

Just as you might have a shower or bath and put on special clothes for an evening out, you may wish to have a similar ritual before you hold circle space. When we prepare for something special, that becomes part of the process and can make the event feel distinctive.

Nervous systems talk to each other and can be particularly affected by the person who is welcoming you into the space and leading the beginning of the process. If the facilitator's sympathetic nervous system is activated, others might subconsciously pick up on this and wonder what the threat is. However, this does not necessarily occur, and it is possible for participants to feel what your intention is (for them to experience something positive) even if you have butterflies in your stomach.

Newcomers may already feel anxious about attending and what will be expected of them. Meeting their arrival having prepared in a way that could enable you to feel calm is therefore helpful. This supports co-regulation where their nervous systems will downregulate to match the calm and grounded feeling that you radiate. Of course, you may feel nervous about running your first circle, but this is different from being stressed out because you're running late or haven't checked whether the venue is suitable for the circle and do not have enough space for everyone.

Sometimes life happens and you may feel anything but self-regulated. Depending on the severity of the situation, it might be that you either need to share this upfront so that people can understand what is happening for you or even cancel/postpone the gathering. If a circle is mature and there are people who attend who have developed their own capacity of holding the space, asking for their support is another option.

People often understand if you state simply and clearly what's happened, such as that there was lots of traffic or you are feeling nervous for a particular reason. If you are clear and calm in the way you share, that makes a difference. Circumstances where you may need to cancel a circle would be ones where you feel that you are unable to settle or may become very emotional. Life happens and sometimes events out of our control mean that the sensible decision is to postpone.

Finding a form of supervision and peer support is helpful, and will be discussed in Chapter 10 along with other ways to support yourself and deepen your facilitation: 'The more I go within myself, the more my work deepens and the more I am able to hold in community... We have to do the work within before we can hold the space' (Tanya Forgan).

Facilitators may have different ways to decide what the circle topic will be:

> I begin with channelling on the day of the circle. I connect to events happening in the world or what I or others are experiencing and write a meditation practice on that theme. The rest of the framing of the circle is the same each week.
>
> *Henika Patel*

> I planned the circles by staring into space and imagining, writing notes by hand, and typing on the laptop. I needed to dig deep to excavate the topics my heart wanted to share... I read a lot, and brought aspects of workshops, retreats and professional trainings I'd attended.
>
> *Julia Paulette Hollenbery*

We often include current events in our circle work, such as the contentious and difficult issues of Britain's vote to leave the EU, abortion rights, the Covid pandemic and the Ukrainian war. While a circle might be about creating a space away from everyday life, it can be important to acknowledge the big events that are affecting people. Bringing big issues into talking circles can also bring about change – for example, a choice to actively do something to improve green spaces in a local area or work in a homeless winter shelter. Some circles are created specifically to raise awareness and bring about activities to help local communities in need.

The circles created could be galvanised to effect positive change. How much time is spent in a circle on sharing experiences about sudden national or global events can be decided together, and extra time on settling and integrating practices would be recommended. In fact, some circles are created with the specific aim of talking about difficult or taboo issues (e.g. a grief circle).

Pacing yourself and putting self-care into place is important to make running circles sustainable. If you are choosing to run a circle addressing a challenging issue, you may need extra training or to put specific safeguards in place, so you do not burn out or experience vicarious trauma. If your intention for the talking circle is to result in taking action, additional attention will be required, and you are likely to need the support of others.

The charity TreeSisters created the concept of Groves: local circles where people were encouraged to effect positive environmental local change. Groves involve a considerable amount of work both to set up and then to create the community work around them – they are not a small undertaking – and as the organisation is a charity, this considerable work would not involve payment. Circles of this kind can work brilliantly.

In Julia's local area, a circle of like-minded individuals created a community wildlife space that is now maintained by volunteers. Careful reflection on the resources you have available might determine whether you charge for a circle, ask for donations or run it for free. Being able to afford what supports you, whether that's good-quality food, services like reflexology or massage, or having supervision with a counsellor, needs to be factored in. Pricing will be considered in more detail in Chapter 18. Charging can also be a sign of commitment to running the circle:

> I never set out to create a business at all. That was not my intention. I charged for circles from day one because I wanted to declare that I felt serious about holding this and I wanted people to take the spaces seriously.
>
> *Stephanie*

Communicating with participants beforehand

The preparation actually begins well before the day of the circle, before settling yourself and setting up the space. Communicating what to expect in the circle will help potential attendees feel more at ease: for example, the basic structure of the event, the timings, that phones are to be switched off and whether there is anything to bring (like a cushion, blanket, mug). This description of the circle starts with your marketing of the event, which we will cover in detail in Chapter 17. Clear details of the address, parking arrangements and public transport are important.

Before the online circle, Henika Patel sends an email inviting her participants to 'shower or bathe, wear something that makes you feel wonderful, bring something that helps you feel connected'. The preparation creates a sense of anticipation and that something special is about to happen. See Chapter 17 for an example email with confirmation/joining instructions.

You might choose to communicate the guidelines and values of your circle prior to people attending. Kate Codrington shares:

> The 'contract' started very early. I spoke about community and about being present with what is. Listening, being present for yourself and for other people. In the emails there was always stuff about turning off your mobile phone: trying to make sure you had an uninterrupted space.

Tessa once had a regular participant of her women's circle bring her young au pair. She thought that the circle would be good for her and help her feel less isolated. There was a language barrier, and it became apparent that the participant hadn't explained to the au pair that people would take it in turns to talk and she wouldn't be able to help interpret. Two-thirds of the way through the circle, the au pair got out her phone and started scrolling. This was a good lesson in making sure that people know what to expect and can decide whether it's something they're interested in.

When one person is organising the circle, there is unseen work in planning, communicating with people, organising the venue, setting up and taking down the space. Although you will benefit from the circle, the time and effort involved must be factored in when deciding whether you need support or how much to charge (i.e. not just for the time of facilitating the circle but the work around it).

Hold your nerve! When holding your first circle, you may find it takes time for people to decide to come. Although some circle holders find the numbers far exceed their expectations, it is common for circles to start with low numbers and build. If it seems likely that the numbers will be small, remember small numbers can give you the opportunity to hone your skills as a circle holder. Eight to 12 people is often seen as the 'perfect number' for a talking circle of between one and two hours, but four to five people could be a really lovely number to start with.

If you cancel a circle because of a small number of participants, those who have taken the time to commit and join you may feel uncertain the second time around. Part of running a circle is proving yourself to be reliable, and that means commitment to running the event even if the numbers are smaller than you imagined. That is another reason why it is worth taking time to consider finances, as it could cost a specific amount to hire a venue and you might feel resentful if you are out of pocket after taking the time and effort to create a circle. (We will discuss money in more detail in Chapter 18.)

Reconnecting with your intentions for the circle

Now all the setting up, settling and communicating is done and you're waiting for the first person to come through the door. Take a moment to reconnect with your intentions. This might be remembering the values or principles that you want to guide all the circles that you do, such as compassion, integrity and authenticity. Or it might be specific to the circle that you're about to hold: why did you want to bring these people together? What did you hope to achieve? Pausing and bringing these intentions to mind brings presence to what you are about to do.

One practice might be to stand in the middle of the circle, face each of the seats one by one and bow (or nod or bring your hands together) to offer your service and humility. You may develop a simple ritual to mark your preparation, such as having a spray to mist over you or some simple words that you repeat. If you collaborate with others, you could sit together for a moment in silence to collect your thoughts and be fully present.

However you choose to prepare, the most important quality is that it feels authentic to you. Take a deep breath; people are about to arrive and the circle to start.

● EXERCISE: 'EVEN' BREATHING

One simple practice for becoming centred and grounded is 'even breathing'. The inhalation and exhalation are of equal length, which means that you are likely to become relaxed but stay alert. Breathe in for a count of five or six seconds and breathe out for the same amount, making sure not to force the breath.

Some people are uncomfortable with the idea of counting the breath, so an alternative would be to breathe in with the focus travelling up the spine and breathe out with the focus travelling back down, or placing one hand on the heart and another at the belly and slowly moving the bottom hand to join the top one at the heart with the in-breath and back down to the belly with the out-breath.

Another alternative is to use arm movement – both hands begin at the chest, and with the in-breath the arms go out to the side and with the out-breath they return to the chest. Each of us has a particular relationship to the breath, and some find it much easier to connect than others. Only do what feels comfortable and easy for you. Continue for a few minutes if you find this useful to bring about a sense of calm.

Julia and Tessa train yoga teachers in practices that involve holding space. Very common feedback from yoga teachers embarking upon circle holding for the first time is that they felt unease and worry about holding the space, even when they have prepared and given themselves time to settle. It is totally okay to feel nervous, and the people in your circle may not even notice. You will find ways of settling that feel right for you. We are sharing ideas, not rules, and hope some of the tips in this chapter have helped.

● EXERCISE: SETTING UP YOUR CIRCLE

Give yourself 20 minutes and have a notepad and coloured pens. Close your eyes and give yourself a few moments to centre yourself. Read each question and after each one take time to reflect. Use the section of the exercise above where you connect to your heart, and give yourself a few breaths with each question before you draw or write your response.

- ● How would you like the circle space to feel?

- ● What can you physically do to create the right atmosphere?

- ● How will you take a moment to settle before everyone arrives?

- How will you shape the participants' expectations of the circle?

- What do you need to tell them ahead of the event?

Now we turn from setting up to how to open your talking and listening circle in the next chapter.

CHAPTER 6

The Importance of Welcoming

Whether it is a short or long journey to get to the place where the talking circle is held, stepping over the threshold is an emotionally charged moment. The courage and curiosity to attend the first time may be the result of months of contemplation and weighing up. For those that have attended before, it can be a moment of relief as people join their tribe of like-minded souls and the longing to belong is met. Being received warmly is everything.

How you welcome people to your circle is so important that it has a chapter of its own. Now that the preparation is done, your attention can be focused on welcoming people into the space you've created. Being at the threshold of the space to say, 'Hello, how's your journey been?' helps people immediately feel valued and that they have a place here. Whether online or in person, your welcome matters. You can put people at ease with a smile and a warm welcome. Ensure that before the start any newcomer is aware of the guidelines and principles of the circle. We will discuss these in more detail in Chapter 8.

> I remember arriving at a circle for the first time. I walked into the hall and some people were already sat in a circle. I wasn't sure who the host was, but then I noticed there was a lady who looked like she was trying to make eye contact with me and smile. The person she was talking to was in the middle of saying something and the host waved me over. As soon as she warmly said, 'Welcome,' I felt myself relax.
>
> *Jemma*

Time is needed for this part of the circle. If you have planned for a 7.30 p.m. start, it is helpful to give people advance warning to arrive 10–15 minutes early to allow time for arriving and feeling settled for the start. Music can be played: you might have attended an event before and noticed that music has added to the ambiance of an event before it has started. Maybe you have decided to put snacks out or offer people a cup of tea. Nerves are usual when people arrive at a setting for the first time, so think about what might put them at ease and give them the time they need to settle and find a comfortable seat.

Show them where they can put shoes and coats, bags and paraphernalia, and where they can sit. If you're having refreshments, offer to get them something or to help themselves. If it's a regular circle or you have a collaborator, you can always delegate someone to do part of this to make it easier for you. Explain where the toilet is if they've never been to the venue before.

Introduce people to each other as they arrive so they can start getting to know someone else and feel more comfortable in the space. If this is a regular meeting, you can assign a new person to someone who is well established in the circle so they are made to feel comfortable. Perhaps you have things out to look at – for example, books about menopause for a menopause circle or about grief for a grief circle. You can direct people to look at those resources so they have something to do instead of feeling awkward. Or perhaps you ask children to bring something special with them and guide them to add it to a curiosity table, with the reassurance that they will be taking them back home later.

Sometimes it can be difficult to juggle welcoming everyone with other people's needs. For example, someone might start telling you an involved story of something that happened since the last circle. In this case, it's important to say something like 'I'm interested to hear about this. Could you share it in the circle or wait until after the circle to tell me? It's important to welcome everyone into the space.'

Csilla Dulàcska shared that for her mum and daughter circles she would contact each mum before the event. They would have a brief conversation on the phone to check in, and this would make her feel less nervous about running the circle because they were no longer strangers and there was less chance of surprises (e.g. major relationship issues between the mum and daughter).

This type of check-in can also be a good opportunity to find out about people's expectations and explain what happens in a circle setting. Csilla says, 'Having a brief phone call beforehand puts the attendees at ease and

ME at ease! I get nervous, but if I've already chatted to people, I can focus on welcoming them and not my nerves.'

Preparing people in advance is useful. It is worth creating a welcome email that can be tailored to individuals so that those attending are well prepared. We will be sharing examples of invitations and welcome letters in Chapter 17. Please feel free to jump to that chapter if you would like help with this now.

Venues in nature like yurts in a field can be a very special place to run circles, but can also be hard to find. Tessa used to run her women's circle in such a place, down narrow lanes in the countryside. It was a glorious space on the edge of a wood that felt very special. In the winter, though, it could be harder to find in the dark evenings. One night, there was fog and she wondered if anybody would arrive at all:

> One by one these figures emerged out of the fog and slipped into the yurt. Two friends had decided to come for the first time that night and the taxi driver wondered where on earth they were going. He wanted to turn back, but they persisted. I gave everyone a warm welcome and a warm mug of tea. There was the most wonderful sense of arrival for that circle.

Julia likes the security of venues with amenities. This is especially import-ant if you want your circles to be inclusive. Is there disabled parking? What is the access like? Are there suitable toilet facilities? Julia often uses her studio for circle gatherings: it is accessible without steps and with easy access to a ground-level toilet and hot water for drinks. It is also in a quiet setting where birdsong is common, and near to fields and a brook so that those who wish to step into nature can do so easily.

Starting on time

Our advice is that you make it clear in communications that there is a start time and it is important to be there for the beginning of the circle (or state how much before attendees can arrive). You can explain the importance of being present for the opening as people introduce themselves and for the guidelines for the talking circle. Otherwise, time will be needed to go over these again and it can be frustrating for those who were present at the start. This is what marks a talking circle as a different kind of gath-ering to an informal meet-up where people come and go or the rules for communication are unspoken.

From a practical point of view, make sure instructions on how to get to a venue and where to park are clear. We ensure that we have their contact details and they have ours, so they can inform us if for any reason they are running late or, if it is the first time they are joining a circle, they have any issues finding the venue or, if driving, parking. You can also ask people to wait until a specific time to come to the door as you will be setting up. It is helpful for you to have access to the venue in good time so that you have both preparation time and time for early arrival.

Your policy on latecomers might depend on what type of circle you're running. You can choose whether you have a hard start time or are flexible. This may also be dictated by the nature of the circle. It's very important that if you have a hard start time, you make it absolutely clear that people arriving beyond the start time will not be admitted to prevent a difficult situation.

For example, you might decide to hold a circle with a theme that is likely to bring up challenging emotions, such as baby loss. If someone were to arrive 30 minutes late, it might be that someone is in the middle of telling their difficult experience and it would be disruptive to bring the new person in. For the person sharing, they might feel uncomfortable about continuing without a sense of who this is from the introductions. For the latecomer, it might feel overwhelming to walk into an emotionally charged space. However, you might honour the courage that it's taken to attend and want to welcome in latecomers. Having a helper who can answer the door, explain what's happened so far and wait for the right moment to bring the person into the circle could make the difference. You need to decide what is right for this particular circle.

If you allow for a soft start with latecomers, it can be helpful to ensure everyone has had the opportunity to discover and agree to the guidelines. If confidentiality is important for your circle, everyone needs to know that and be in agreement.

This is another reason why the invitation is important, because it will set the scene for everyone involved if you have shared the guidelines ahead of the gathering. One of the reasons people are nervous about attending a talking circle is that it is an unusual way of communicating: the conventional rules of society do not apply. It is therefore important that the guidelines of attending a circle are understood as this will put the participants at ease.

Once everyone is seated, you could make eye contact with each participant in the circle to help them feel welcomed and seen. In cases where your circle is taking place in the evening around a campfire, eye contact is not necessary. If the gathering is round a fire in a dark evening, there is likely to be less formality to the gathering.

● EXERCISE: JUGGLING PEOPLE'S NEEDS

Read through this example and identify what issues could arise. Reflect on how you could set things up differently to support everyone's needs.

> You arrive and ring the doorbell. There's no answer and you wonder if you've got the right time. After a while, the host opens the door and apologises that she was setting things up in the garden.
>
> The circle is run on a collaborative basis. Most people know each other and so there is a friendly, warm welcome. It's a hot summer evening so the host suggests having the circle outside in the garden. A space is cleared and those that have shawls put them down over the grass. The garden is overlooked and the neighbour's windows are wide open because of the heat.
>
> A couple of people are missing, but everyone present agrees to start the circle. The introductions are followed by a beautiful meditation. The guidelines and the topic to talk about are explained. Three-quarters of an hour into the two-hour circle, the host's phone goes off because the doorbell can't be heard in the garden. The host disappears to let the two latecomers in. She's gone for ten minutes, and when they come into the circle, the men say they were running late because they stopped to buy drinks to bring.
>
> The introductions are repeated. Mosquitos start to appear and so the host goes into the house to get citronella candles. Someone apologises and says they're going to go now because they've been bitten and are feeling uncomfortable. Another person sneezes and complains that early evening is a time when the pollen count is at its height and the dimming sun is shining right into their eyes. The host sees them out and, in the meantime, the talking turns to chatting. It turns into a social gathering and some stay well beyond the two hours.

Take a moment to write down your thoughts about the preparation, welcome and set up of the circle. What issues might there be? What changes could you make?

Of course, unexpected things in life happen, like late buses, and people will arrive late from time to time. If someone habitually arrives late, it's advisable to talk to them and understand why. If you have started to set expectations before the day of the event on when to arrive, you will have fewer distractions as the facilitator and can focus on welcoming.

The container that is created is special and starts with the welcome into the space. It is okay to have clear guidelines that explain that latecomers will not be permitted. It is also okay to bend those rules if appropriate.

There are definitely circle situations which do not require a hard start, like parent and child circles, some embodiment circles and circles that are less formal and involve crafts. In these cases, we would recommend gently repeating the guidelines for newcomers and inviting them to take their time to settle.

EXERCISE: PLANNING YOUR WELCOME

Remember or imagine what it feels like to be welcomed: when have you felt most comfortable being welcomed, and when most uncomfortable?

Now imagine this for your circle, with your particular attendees in mind. Here are some questions to help your reflection:

- Would a hard or soft start time work best? (A specific arrival time with a cut-off or an open door?)

- How might it work with regular participants as opposed to brand-new ones?

- Have you created space and time for newcomers to arrive early so they can feel more settled before the start of the circle? (Or don't have to stand outside in the rain if their bus arrived early?)

- Would you like there to be a specific amount of time for informal gathering and greeting before the start of circle? (Or would it be better at the end? Why? Have you accounted for that time in your schedule and venue hire?)

- If it's an online circle, will you set up a waiting room and let everyone in at the same time? (More on this in Chapter 16.)

- How are you creating an ambiance for the welcome part of the circle? (Music, refreshments, resources to look at.)

- How do you balance sharing logistical information (e.g. where the fire exits are, to turn off mobile phones) with a warm, personable welcome?

Now that we have welcomed people into the circle space, the next chapter shares examples of opening practices that can be included before the talking and listening get under way.

CHAPTER 7

Opening and Settling

Everyone has found a place to sit and there is an air of anticipation.
In the centre of the circle is a centrepiece that draws the eye and
signals that this is not a normal gathering for chit-chat. Something
special may happen here today. Settling is needed to soothe nervous
systems activated by the journey to get here or everyday busy-ness.
Time is given to fully arrive at this moment.

If you like, close your eyes after reading this sentence, take a slow breath in and out, connect with now.

The process of opening the circle is all about setting the scene. It can be done in different ways and we're going to give you a variety of examples. We recommend pausing before you launch into the official opening process. Take a moment to smile, look around the circle and connect with everyone's eyes. Scanning the circle, you might say, 'Welcome to this circle. I'm so happy you're here.'

You can also have set words written down that you repeat every circle. Repeated behaviours can form part of the feeling of belonging, create familiarity and soothe the nervous system if they are chosen well. People often enjoy ritual and may remember it fondly from childhood: from saying grace before a meal to taking the register at school.

Ritual can be something that is lost later in life, and the grounding nature of this may have been very comforting. You can find words that support people to become present or fit your intention for your circle. For example:

All that I am is welcome to be.
All that I hear is welcome to be.
All that I feel is welcome to be.
Just as it is.

Another example, if the four elements are relevant to your circle, is that you could invite everyone to face the four points of the compass while repeating words such as:

> Earth to the North, I honour you, hail and welcome!
> Air to the East, I honour you, hail and welcome!
> Fire to the South, I honour you, hail and welcome!
> Water to the West, I honour you, hail and welcome!

(Repeat after the circle with 'hail and farewell' to each direction.)

Another way to use words to open the circle might be to choose a relevant poem. Favourite books of ours for this purpose are John O'Donohue's *Benedictus*, Ana Sampson's *She Is Fierce: Brave, Bold and Beautiful Poems by Women*, Lorin Roche's *The Radiance Sutras*, Lalla's *Naked Song* (translated by Coleman Barks), Jeff Foster's *The Way of Rest*, William Sieghart's *The Poetry Pharmacy* and stories from Clarissa Pinkola Estés' *Women Who Run with Wolves*.

THE HEART
The heart is an unlimited room.
There is always enough room
for the contents of this moment.
The highest joy,
the deepest agony,
thoughts that won't stop spinning,
the heart can hold it all.
Embrace is all it knows.
Space is its nature.
It needs no time.
It asks nothing.
It gives everything in return.

(*Excerpt from 'The Heart', in* The Way of Rest, *permission granted by Jeff Foster.*)

Sharing a poem or reading can create a reflective tone to the sharing space. In this poem, the heart could be replaced by the circle and it would be perfectly fitting.

Your circle may have precepts or guidelines that are recited each time you gather. Depending on what kind of initial introductions and check-ins you are planning, we would suggest leaving the explanation of these and the etiquette for the circle until later. For example, if you plan something simple to start, such as for people to say their name and one sentence about how they are today, it allows everyone to use their voice and to feel welcome before the deeper talk starts. Circle guidelines will be covered in the next chapter.

Lighting a candle can be a symbolic way to mark the formal start of a circle. Making a simple sound such as striking a hand chime three times can also bring a sense of ritual or occasion. It can also be used if people have been busy chatting to each other while waiting for the circle to begin, to get their attention.

Introductions and initial check-in

The initial round of talking helps people to settle into the circle and find their voice. It's similar to how on the radio a presenter will ask a brief question of all the speakers. Otherwise, the person to be interviewed last will be sitting and waiting for a while, perhaps feeling trepidation or anxiety. There is also something fundamental in saying your name out loud in a circle that makes people feel witnessed.

We recommend that the initial introduction and check-in are kept simple: make it as easy as possible to answer with a simple question that is not loaded with emotion. You could invite people to share their name and what has brought them to circle today in one sentence. If you want to start with a short check-in, asking for people to share one word or two words for how they feel in the moment can be practical.

Tessa phrases it like this: 'I would like you to give two words for how you feel right now; you don't need to explain why you feel that way and they might be opposites. It's also okay if you don't know how you feel.' Then the facilitator starts with their two words to model how it's done. It's helpful to share the information yourself first so that you're modelling what to do.

Being asked something as seemingly simple as 'How are today?' can be difficult and could immediately put someone in the position of not wishing to share information. Perhaps they are finding their feelings challenging or are feeling something they don't think is okay, or maybe they are not sure how they feel.

Julia loves the practice of welcoming people into the circle using their name, repeating 'Welcome [Name]' for each person. She invites each person to say their name and then everyone welcomes them by their name into the circle. Although this is a simple practice, there is something very special about being acknowledged by your name. Also, because the person themselves is invited to say their name first, if there is any confusion around pronunciation, the fact they have said it themselves first will help everyone in the group pronounce their name correctly.

With children, a simple icebreaker might be to ask for their name and favourite flavour of ice cream, if they like it. For a circle with a menstrual cycle awareness focus, you might ask people to share where they are in their cycle, with an explanation of how Day 1 corresponds to the first day of their period, and that it's okay if they don't know where they are, don't currently have a cycle or don't want to share. For a parents' group, asking people to share their own name and the name and age of the child gives an identity to the parent too!

There can be ways of bringing a sense of ceremony into the check-in where this is appropriate for your circle. For example, you could set up a round mirror as part of the centrepiece, with a large candle in the middle surrounded by tealight candles, with one tealight for each person present. As each person says their name, they light their own candle and then repeat this phrase 'With this candle, I call myself fully present.' At the end of the circle, part of the closing can be people blowing out their own candle.

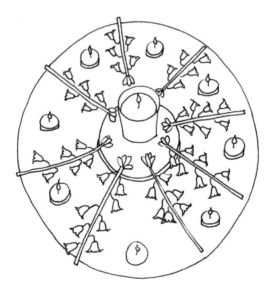

Figure 7.1 Mandala on mirror with bluebells and tealight candles

It might be appropriate to make a physical gesture like bringing the palms together for the namaste greeting in a yoga setting. There is often a level of expectation that hand mudras will be used and that Sanskrit terms will be used too. If the decision is made to do this, then it is appropriate for this to be done with cultural sensitivity to the tradition it comes from.

● EXERCISE: SEASONAL CHECK-IN

When welcoming people to circle, Julia often uses the seasons. When newcomers attend, she gives a short explanation and gives them the opportunity to speak last so they have seen how the welcome works. Using this seasonal reference is especially useful in embodiment circles where there may be a physical practice as part of the gathering, as it gives the facilitator an idea of energy levels in the room.

This is how you can explain the seasons:

Winter:

- Possibly feeling tired, getting over an illness, maybe hasn't slept well the night before.

- Equates with the external season of winter and the need to rest.

- Connects to the time of the bleed. (There are certain physical practices which can be helpful at this time and others less so, so this would give Julia an indication of what might be appropriate in the movement part of the gathering.)

Spring:

- Could relate to a feeling of shyness or cheekiness.

- Connects to the external season of spring – in the Western hemisphere this might mean lots of spring flowers and mixed weather. Lighter skies.

- Relates to being a young child or a teenager in the life cycle.

Summer:

- Some might love the summer and might relate to a feeling of being full of energy, feeling fantastic, full of life and vigour.

- Others might not love the summer and equate this season to a feeling of overwhelm; perhaps too many hours of sunshine, not enough rest.

- Equates with the ovulation phase of the menstrual cycle.

Autumn:

- Equates with maybe feeling out of sorts, annoyed, or feeling a need for clearing things out and completion.

- Option you can choose if you have no idea how you feel.

- Connects to the pre-menstruum in the menstrual cycle.

It is also fine for people to respond with a mix of the seasons. In Julia's circles, there are often people present who do not have a menstrual cycle and/or never had one and they are still very happy to join in! This connection between the 'Inner Seasons' of the menstrual cycle and the 'Outer Seasons' are based on Red School's work on menstruality.

A speaking object can also be introduced here (see the section 'Creating the right atmosphere' in Chapter 5). This object marks whose turn it is to speak. This could be a decorated stick, a bowl or something that fits with your theme. You could create the tradition of everyone bringing their own special item to the circle to be used in this way, and invite them to state when they are done or what they have said is at an end. They could finish with something simple like 'I have spoken.'

The order of introductions, settling and giving guidelines is not set in stone. Reflect on what supports the needs of the people in your circle best. You also have the option to have a settling practice before introductions to give people the opportunity to settle their nervous system before speaking. We suggest not asking people to close their eyes for a settling practice until the introductions have been done, so they feel comfortable with who is in the room.

Using a settling practice

Either before or after the initial check-in and introductions, it may feel more comfortable for people to close their eyes for a settling practice or do some movement less self-consciously. Always give people the option to keep their eyes open as some people are more comfortable with this. You can invite them to lower or soften their gaze instead.

The settling practice may take as little as 2–5 minutes or be a much bigger part of the gathering depending on what your intention is. The purpose of the settling practice is to allow people's nervous systems to downregulate and move into the alert relaxation state, which is more conducive to talking and sharing. It can be as simple as inviting people to take a deep breath in and sigh or yawn as they breathe out, and repeating this three times.

What settling practice you use may depend on what skills you have. For example, if you are a yoga or meditation teacher, you might use techniques from your classes. You could also use a script or a recording of a meditation if you are not confident at leading one when you first start facilitating. There are apps like Insight Timer that have free meditations where you can set the length of time. (Check the legal requirements if you choose to share something that is not of your own creation. With music and meditation there are specific laws depending on where you live.)

If you are using a relaxation or meditation script, familiarise yourself with it beforehand and try the practice yourself. Be aware of the pace and modulation of your voice. Slowing down, lowering your voice and having less modulation (without becoming monotone) will support people to settle.

● EXERCISE: EXAMPLES OF SETTLING PRACTICES

Here are some examples of what Tessa and Julia use in their circles.

Embodiment practice

You might wish to words such as these:

> Get comfortable, leaning back into the support of the chair if you can. You can have your eyes open or closed. Take a moment to feel the contact between your back and the support. Take your awareness down your legs and to your feet. Maybe wiggle your toes as you bring your awareness from the head and all the way down to your toes.

> Become aware of your breath. You do not need to change it, but perhaps you want to take a longer breath in and sigh out. Yawns are welcome. Have a sense of your body in the room, in this circle of people. You might feel that your body is ready to rest a bit more, with your shoulders dropping away from your ears, or your legs and feet feeling heavier.

> Take a few moments to make a space to check in with yourself. What is alive for you right now? Is there something you might want to share today to feel seen and heard? How would it be to feel supported in this circle?

Become aware of the room around you again. Open your eyes a little to let light in, if your eyes aren't already open. You might want to move and stretch or change position.

Resting practice

If you are in a venue with a space to rest and you have set an expectation that restful practices could be part of the gathering, starting with the opportunity to rest can be a beautiful way to begin.

You can use words like these:

Lie down in a comfortable position and allow your attention to come to your breathing. Feel free to have the eyes either open or closed. As you bring your attention to your breath, you might notice the coolness of the air as it enters through your nostrils. You could be aware that the air that leaves feels different – possibly warmer than the air entering.

Notice how comfortable or not it is to breathe in and out through the nostrils. If mouth breathing is more comfortable, then do that.

Allow your attention to come down to your body. Trace the attention from your heels up to the top of your head. Trace your attention back down from the top of your head to the tips of your toes. Continue with this practice for a little while. [Pause]

Allow your attention to come back to your breathing. Bring your knees into your tummy and rock from side to side (NB this is not appropriate with pregnancy) and roll over to one side.

Come up to a comfortable sitting position. Allow yourself to re-orientate yourself in the room. Maybe look up to the sky/ceiling, to your left and right and to the ground. Notice your sit bones beneath you and notice the presence of other people in the room.

Reading practice

Sharing someone else's words to create the right tone can be helpful. Introduce the words something like this: 'Settle down in a comfortable seated or lying position. I am going to read you a short story/poem. You can listen as much or as little as you like to the story. Once it is complete, we will come into a circle together.'

At this point, you can introduce a story or poem that connects to the theme of your circle.

Senses practice

You can use words like this to connect people with their senses:

> Let's connect with the present moment and start to let go of the busy-ness of the day. Get as comfortable as you can. Have a look around the room and name silently three things you can see. [Pause] If you feel comfortable, now close your eyes and listen. [Pause] Name silently up to three things you can hear. Then, name three things you can physically feel. [Pause] Notice how you've come into the present moment by using your senses.
>
> Imagine that you're sitting with a good friend. You feel comfortable sitting quietly together. You're making space for if something wants to be shared. You're here together, sitting companionably. As you create space, perhaps a feeling, image or thought appears. Imagine your friend has shared it with you and you're waiting to see what else comes up, rather than going off into your own story.
>
> Perhaps nothing comes up and it's okay to sit quietly, enjoying the space to simply be.
>
> If something stronger comes up, rather than merging completely with the emotion, see if you can stay on the edge of it. You can think, 'A part of me feels...' so that it doesn't overwhelm you.
>
> Perhaps you could try this phrase: 'No wonder I feel...because...' to bring self-compassion and self-kindness. For example, 'No wonder I feel tired because I've had a busy day.'
>
> Now become aware of your body again. Be aware of the room around you and open your eyes if they are closed. Have a look around and remind your-self where you are. If it's helpful, name three things that you can see to bring you into the present again.

This can be a helpful settling practice to get in touch with feelings and intro-duce ideas to support those who tend to get overwhelmed.

● EXERCISE: MEDITATION PRACTICE WITH THE SENSES

This is slightly different to the practice above because it is less directive.

> Notice the cool air entering and the warm air leaving. Allow your attention to come to your nose. Is it possible to notice your sense of smell? With each in-breath, connect with your sense of smell. Is it possible to identify a smell?

Maybe your own perfume or soap. Or have you noticed a particular smell from this room? Or from outside of this room?

As you focus on your sense of smell, do you notice that what you can smell changes each time you breathe in? Or does it remain the same? Are you aware of a moment in time when you are able to notice smell? When you breathe out, do you notice that the sense of smell is not active?

You could introduce the senses of touch and hearing in a similar way.

If you are relying on your voice alone for a settling practice, it is important to notice the pace and tone with which you speak. The first time you run a circle, you might be nervous, so we recommend practising on friends and family before sharing a meditation practice or something that is not familiar to you as there are easier ways to open a circle.

If you come to circle holding with a pre-existing skill – for example, as a meditation or yoga teacher or musician – you might find that choosing to use that particular skill in settling can be the easiest option. Keep it simple and short, and as you become more familiar with settling practices, you can become more adventurous.

Using movement to settle

Movement can be a wonderful way to help people move away from their everyday awareness or feelings of nervousness to a more embodied, calmer state. The movement practice can be simple and still effectively soothe the nervous system. If you don't have much space, you can remain seated. It could be as simple as: stretching up towards the ceiling, one hand at a time; interlacing the fingers and pushing the palms away; circling the ankles; alternating pointing the toes with pushing the heels away. If it feels appropriate, you could introduce rhythmic arm movements connected with the inhalation or exhalation.

Depending on your skills, yoga, tai chi or dance movements could be used to help people move away from their everyday awareness to a more embodied state. If this is a longer section of the circle, it would be important to communicate this with people in advance so that they wear appropriate clothing and can share any contraindications for movement with you. Being clear about what activities will happen at the event will prevent surprises and people feeling uncomfortable.

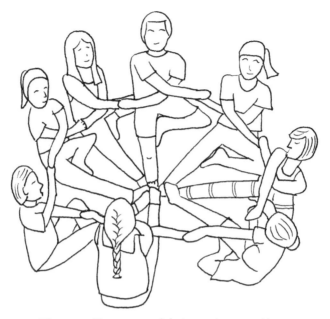

Figure 7.2 Human mandala to create connection

Shaking

Movement can also be used later in the circle to provide a break from talking. This is especially useful if strong emotions have arisen and the circle is 'stuck' in them, or if a disagreement has arisen and is hard to move on from. Shaking is an excellent practice for these situations as it can be done gently or vigorously depending on how a person feels.

Invite everyone to stand and find space (perhaps behind their chair depending on how your venue is set up). Starting with the arms, imagine shaking the hands off the ends of the arms. Shift the weight to one foot and shake the other leg as if shaking the foot off the end of it. Shift the weight to the other foot and repeat. You can use the whole body in the shaking movement until it feels like anything that was stuck has had a chance to move.

Havening

Another lovely somatic technique is havening. Literally, this is creating your own haven. Cross your arms over your chest so that you have a hand on the opposite upper arm as if you are giving yourself a hug. Stroke the hands down the arms towards the elbows slowly, choosing gentle or firmer pressure. Continue with the movement, or pause, hugging the arms into your body. The touch can enable oxytocin to flow, and this generates a feeling of wellbeing. In a new circle where people don't know each other, havening can be a lovely way of providing touch without infringing personal space!

After opening the circle and sharing a settling practice, you might want to check in again to see whether people are comfortable and how the settling practice was received. Then you're ready to share or co-create the guidelines/values for the circle.

A short settling practice

If your time is limited, it is possible to run a circle without a settling practice. We have attended circles that have not included this and have gone straight into a short share. However, even if you have one or two minutes, it can be nice to honour the start of your circle in a way that can help people manage their nerves (something that is very common at the start of a circle). If time is an issue, maybe inviting people to notice how they are sitting, look around the room and smile at each other can be a simple, short way to begin.

When the setting influences settling practices

If you decide that a campfire or some other kind of fire works well as your centrepiece, you could start the circle with every participant adding a piece of wood to the fire. If you're in a beautiful setting, you can invite people to look outside and to the horizon.

When you're running a circle in a busy, noisy place like a festival, it's important to draw attention to the distractions rather than ignore that they're there. You can acknowledge the environment, saying that part of the person will be aware of those noises and another part can focus on being part of the circle.

Music as settling practice

It might be that you choose to have a specific song or chant that fits with the theme of your circle. It could be a simple song that people who join can easily learn. Having a song to start each circle can be an easy way to start and gives people the opportunity to use their voices before taking the step of speaking alone.

Some people do not enjoy singing or chanting, so inviting everyone to either join in or participate through listening allows this practice to be inclusive. As simple a song or chant as possible would be recommended, with a close connection to the focus of your group. We share examples of songs and chants in Chapter 11. Inviting people to dance with their eyes closed can help prevent them from feeling shy or embarrassed. Invite them to stand, take a couple of breaths and move to the music.

Music can be used both in welcoming and settling (ensure that you have legal permission). You can invite people to come in and begin to dance to the music that is played. If you have little time for settling, the use of music can mix the welcome with the settling, playing music at a low level as people arrive and then slowly turning it right down and then off to begin the circle.

If this all sounds a bit serious or complicated, Benedict Beaumont has some advice:

> People do need to go to those deep places but also need to be reminded about how joyful life can be. That fun side of us. Not just permissible to have fun but it can also be celebrated and normalised. We can play like children.

> Introducing music can bring joy and fun into circles – we are allowed to be foolish and get it wrong and just have a laugh. I often start with the idea, shall we just have some fun today? Lightness, joy and humour allow us to go way deeper – open up more. So I begin with the idea, what can we do to bring in joy?

Benedict often invites people to keep their eyes closed when they dance at the start of his circles. When we can't see each other, it can help us be less inhibited in our dancing. The idea of not being able to dance is lessened or removed when nobody is looking at you moving. He asks people to take a couple of breaths and then begin to move. He might share a piece of pop music that is very familiar and invites movement; for example, Taylor Swift's 'Shake It Off' literally invites people to shake off their worries.

Writing or drawing to settle

You might give people a piece of paper and a pen and set them a short task to write or draw about that will be used as part of the sharing process at the beginning of the circle. Giving time for people to collect their thoughts on a topic before sharing can be helpful. People don't like to be put on the spot! Benedict Beaumont says, 'People hate being awkward and not knowing what to do – if you have a pen and paper and give them a task, it can settle people.'

● EXERCISE: REFLECTING ON OPENING AND SETTLING

Get some paper and a pen to answer these questions:

- How do you plan to mark the beginning of the circle (to make it distinct from welcoming into the space)?
- What skills or resources do you have to support people to settle into the circle?
- Do you plan to include movement or are there specific items to bring? Have you let people know in the marketing?
- If it's a regular circle, will the opening and settling section be the same every time or vary?

We recommend you practise on some friends or speak aloud to yourself to check the timings and flow.

CIRCLE STORY: CREATING CEREMONY

Tessa shares the creation of a wonderful circle container at the Red School Menstruality Leadership training:

> We were asked to wash before coming to the closing circle for the training. We had been told before the residential training to bring something special to wear for the last day. So we all dressed in our finery. There was a growing sense of anticipation.

> We lined up outside the room where the circles had been taking place. Previously, we could come in and out as we wished, so this felt different. Alexandra and Sjanie were putting the finishing touches to the space.

When the door opened, the room had been tidied and decorated. A beautiful centrepiece had been created with a bowl of water that had been left under the night sky the evening before to soak up the moonlight. Beautiful flowers and bowls of Moontime chocolates brought a feeling of specialness.

We were invited to walk in silently and take our places for the final coming together.

We recommend you stick with what you find easiest and what is most familiar. If you don't yet feel comfortable sharing meditation or embodiment practices, have a go with your best friend or family members. See how you feel about sharing the practice and get feedback from those you are sharing the practice with. The simplest settling practices you might start with are 'Havening' and 'A short settling practice', which we hope you don't find too daunting. If you feel totally uncomfortable with settling practices, you could dive straight in without them.

You may not wish to use a settling practice in your circle. It is possible that welcoming, followed by letting people know the structure and guidelines of the circle, is sufficient. Circle time can also be a more organic process. We find that the more familiar we become with the process of circle, the more able we are to adapt for different circumstances.

As a facilitator, I'm gently exploring and going with the group. To be honest, if I don't feel that something is appropriate for the group and it is planned, I won't do it. I make adjustments for who is in the space.

Sophie Cleere

See what works for you and your attendees. Sometimes it is fine to dive straight in, especially if you have set the scene in some other way, such as using music or setting out your circle in a particular way.

There is an art to holding space, which you will become more confident in with practice. While you will have a plan for your talking circle, you will also be able to adapt to those who are there that day and what unfolds.

In the next chapter, we look at how to share guidelines with your circle.

CHAPTER 8

Sharing Your Circle Guidelines

*After the opening and settling, everyone is waiting with antici-
pation for the deeper-level talking and listening to begin. You share
guidelines like confidentiality, respect, non-judgement, inclusion
and taking responsibility for yourself. They're familiar from the
information you shared in publicising the event. The container for
the circle becomes stronger.*

In everyday life, communication is governed by unwritten rules. A conversation may flow happily backwards and forwards without any agenda, or
one person may hog the opportunity to talk. Someone may ask how you
are, but not pause to hear the answer. The other person may constantly
try to fix the issue that you're talking about when you haven't asked for
advice. You might notice that the other person is not really listening to
what you're saying but waiting for the smallest gap to come in and thinking
about what they're going to say next.

Listening is a skill.

> The average person, if they're not trained in active listening, they only lis-
> ten for 17 seconds at a time! Listening is at the cornerstone of everything.
> How do you even receive information if you're not listening? It is hard. It
> is a practice. It's like working out. It's like a muscle.
>
> *Lee Keylock*

Our culture focuses on the talking part of a conversation. Part of what
you are doing in a circle is teaching how to listen deeply and to talk with
awareness. This might be new to some people who attend and will take
practice. What should the circle be called? A talking circle or a listening
circle? Where would you put the emphasis?

The guidelines you set up for your circle will change the way people talk and listen. Framing the session with the circle values will bring about the magic of people listening with their whole selves to others. The muddiness of everyday communication falls away and there is a clarity that all emotions are welcome here. There is no-one who is too much or too quiet.

If you frame the space well, those people who have a tendency in their daily lives to speak more will feel comfortable speaking less and giving space for others. Those who may not feel they have a voice in their daily lives will be more likely to feel comfortable speaking. Framing is the most important aspect of circle holding as it encourages the choice for equal participation, and this helps people share their vulnerabilities and experiences, perhaps for the first time.

While you could introduce the guidelines for the first time at the circle, we recommend you start framing your circle before people even arrive by sharing the values in marketing information about the event and in confirmation emails or joining instructions. If people understand these guidelines before you hold the circle, it is likely they will feel more comfortable about attending. You are also less likely to have people break the guidelines or challenge the harmony of the circle if there is a prior understanding around the framing for the gathering.

If you want your circle to be collaborative and co-created, we suggest meeting to discuss this before you open the circle. If you have a two-hour circle, creating the guidelines and values from scratch could take a considerable proportion of the time. Where you are hosting a day workshop or retreat, creating the precepts could be the topic of the first circle. When we have worked in collaboration with others, one of the first aspects we discuss is the framing of our event and how to share those guidelines with our community.

Introducing the guidelines

It is helpful to clearly explain that we have the guidelines to support meaningful communication. Guidelines or 'framing' should always be explained in a new circle. They can be repeated every time in regular circles as a reminder to new attendees and also because people's understanding of them can change and deepen over time.

It's useful to see the guidelines as something that is flexible within the context of the needs of the group and the timing of your meeting. As the creator of your circle, you take responsibility for framing your circle so that you have created a container that is most likely to fulfil your intention.

In general, the foundations of a healthy talking circle are (these will be described in detail below):

- confidentiality and safeguarding

- respect

- non-judgement

- speaking from 'I' not 'you' or 'we'

- quality of speaking – for example, from the heart, lean speech

- not offering solutions or aiming to fix situations or people

- taking responsibility for yourself

- timekeeping (participants to arrive on time, facilitators to finish on time).

Tessa included 'respecting the space' as a guideline in mother and daughter circles that moved around the attendees' homes month to month. Being in an informal home setting meant that some girls needed a reminder that not everyone is allowed to jump on their sofas! You might be able to think of other guidelines that are specific to the people who attend your circle.

While inclusion is sometimes appropriate to have as a foundational principle, circle gatherings are often supported by a clear description of who they are for and why they are taking place. This means that they are not necessarily inclusive of everyone. If we use the value of being 'inclusive', it is important to reflect on who we are including and excluding. (See the section on inclusivity in circles in Chapter 3.)

Too many so-called safe spaces or people with positions of authority have been proven to not be safe at all. With 'cancel culture' at its peak, it can feel threatening to speak openly for fear of saying something that will offend someone. That is why guidelines are so helpful and creating groups for specific demographics can be exactly what is needed.

Tanya Forgan, who holds spaces for all people and also specifically for people of mixed race/dual heritage, says, 'There were no spaces for me to go because the circles I went to were mainly white women. So for me to bring that piece of work [about race] did not feel safe.' Although the circles Tanya attended were 'brave spaces', she set up her mixed/dual heritage circles so that people of dual and mixed heritage could come and share more comfortably.

The next exercise supports you to think through how you communicate who the circle is for, the need it's fulfilling and which values are useful to share.

● EXERCISE: COMMUNICATING YOUR VALUES

You may choose to codify your guiding principles so that anyone who joins your circle is aware of them, and post them clearly on your website, leaflet or poster.

It is helpful to begin with the aims and objectives of your circle so that people can choose to attend because they understand that it has been created with their needs in mind.

You might begin with information for newcomers:

[Name of circle] is a talking circle of people who share [characteristics, similar experiences].

Requirement for joining: [e.g. a person of dual heritage, someone who has a menstrual cycle, a parent with a child under the age of two, etc.].

The primary purpose of the circle is....

The talking circle starts with checking in and a settling practice. The topic of [name of topic] is then introduced and we listen to each other's reflections and experiences. At the end of the circle, we close with another check-in.

The circle is run by [your name] with support from [co-facilitator's name if there is one]. [If applicable you could explain the experience the people running the circle have if there will be a teaching element, e.g. a meditation circle led by someone who is a trained meditation practitioner, or an LGBTQIA+ embodiment circle led by a yoga therapist from within the LGBTQIA+ community].

The talking circle is run with the values of respect, non-judgement, confidentiality, not providing solutions, and taking responsibility for your own speech and actions.

Sometimes location precludes inclusivity because access issues prevent those with physical differences from attending. The idea of a listening circle can exclude people with hearing challenges by its nature. Our intention is to include everyone. However, this is not always possible. Inclusion is usually a consideration ahead of facilitating the circle rather than a guideline shared during the event: hopefully, those who are present are the intended participants!

Next, we go into more depth on each of the different guidelines. This is not an exclusive list, and we encourage you to read through them with your specific demographic in mind.

Confidentiality and safeguarding

What is said in the circle stays in the circle.

The principle is that you can tell others about what you yourself shared in the circle, but not what others shared. It might feel very tempting to share some fascinating insight or intense experience that you've heard, but it's not yours to share. This is always important, but especially so where people may mutually know others who aren't present.

Depending on the content of the circle or who attends, it may be important to talk about safeguarding in relation to confidentiality. If something is heard within the circle where a person is at risk of harm, the facilitator may have a duty of care to share it with a medic, police officer, teacher or other. This sounds easy and clear cut but isn't always.

Tessa once ran a circle where someone disclosed that they had attempted suicide the night before. During and after the circle, she ascertained what state of mind the person was now in and whether there was a duty of care to act on. In England, you can attend a mental health first aid course to recognise symptoms and know what action to take. Some councils offer free spaces for people working with children on child and young person mental health qualification trainings.

When working with children in the UK, it may be necessary to have a Disclosure and Barring Service (DBS) check. Tessa always has parents/caregivers present in private workshops and teachers present in school talks and still has a DBS check for reassurance. If you are working with children unsupervised, you may need a higher-level check (Enhanced DBS check). It is also usual in these circumstances to have received additional safeguarding training – within youth organisations, safeguarding training is usually a requirement.

Respect and non-judgement

First, some definitions:

- Respect: Having due regard for a person's feelings, wishes and rights.

- Non-judgement: Neither judging nor criticising. Avoid articulating judgements based on your own personal and moral standards.

It is very easy to say that those in the circle should be respectful and non-judgemental, but in practice we can find that we are very challenged. It can be more helpful to suggest that we are aiming to be respectful and non-judgemental and to nurture the ability to notice when this is not happening.

Encouraging and modelling talking from 'I' rather than 'you' or 'we' can help people own what they're saying. For example, 'I can see how differently I parent, and I'd like to understand more about your perspective' enables communication, rather than 'Your way of parenting is wrong.'

Although some topics are more likely to bring up differences of opinion, it is impossible to anticipate where a talking circle may lead. This is not to scare anyone out of facilitating one, but to show the importance of putting the foundations in place so that you can remind people of the guidelines when needed. A calming practice or breaking to make tea can always be used to let emotions settle.

Deeyah Khan is a Muslim woman who made a documentary called *White Right: Meeting the Enemy*. She spent time doing what's been termed 'extreme listening' with white supremacists, trying to understand why they hate people like her. In a few cases, they became friends after she listened non-judgementally and they were able to really see her as another human being.

If you are facilitating a regular circle, respect and non-judgement could be one of the first themes, so that you have space to unpack what this means and how difficult it is to be non-judgemental when our beliefs can be so ingrained.

With younger children, it can be helpful to explain these concepts by talking about the difference between kind and unkind ways of speaking.

In creating brave spaces, we believe it is possible for people to sit in circle and talk with freedom when they hold opposing views. It is the opposite of what we might experience in a political space where the aim is to shoot down another's opinion. Talking circles can be at their best when they give space for understanding between people who may on the surface seem as though they could never have a point of agreement.

Speaking from 'I'

Encouraging people in the circle to talk from 'I' rather than 'you' or 'we' supports people to own their experience and avoid speaking for others' experience. In everyday conversation, however, it's common to use 'you' in a generic way. For example, 'You win some, you lose some.' This is different from addressing a specific person, such as by saying, 'Are you free for lunch tomorrow?'

A study published in *Science* journal by Orvell, Kross and Gelman (2017) found that people often use 'you' to make it easier to talk about a negative experience and provide a bit of distance from it. People also (subconsciously) used 'you' to move beyond their own experience and attempt to make it a situation that others can relate to. In this sense, 'you' obliquely means 'me'.

'We' is another slippery pronoun that can be used ambiguously. In a circle context, it can be unhelpful when it assumes people have something in common. For example, 'We women have a horrible time with periods.' The intention is to be inclusive and create empathy, but it assumes that everyone present has a horrible time when there's likely to be a range of experiences. Another way it can be used is showing affiliation with a group of people, such as 'We will win the league' or 'We won the war'. In both of these scenarios, it's unlikely the person directly contributed to winning the league or the war and takes the speaker away from personal experience.

The reason for explaining this is that in a circle situation, the use of 'you' and 'we' in the ways detailed above can cause confrontation and discomfort. Inviting people to reflect on how they can speak from 'I' shifts how they speak from subconscious patterns into consciously choosing their words.

Don't be surprised if people lapse into 'you' and 'we' as it is such a common mode of speaking and might be making it easier for someone to talk about difficult things. Gently remind the person why we practise speaking with 'I' when it feels appropriate.

An exception might be when the facilitator realises that the people who've spoken so far have all given the same perspective about an experience, which makes it harder for those with a different experience to now come in. For example, in a recent circle, more than half the participants had a difficult experience with a religious upbringing and so Tessa reflected, 'I know of people who take great comfort in their religious background and the community that's provided.' That wasn't her experience so she couldn't talk from 'I', but it meant that a new person was able to share an opposing experience.

Reflecting on the quality of speaking and listening

In addition to the guideline around confidentiality, with what's said in circle staying in circle, there are other helpful norms that you can explain and encourage:

- Speak from the heart (express authentic self rather than what you think others want to hear).

- Listen from the heart (listening with an open mind and an attitude of compassion).

- When others speak, do not start thinking about how to respond but listen fully.

- Speak spontaneously (express what is happening for you now rather than what you thought you might speak about before the circle began).

- Lean speech (focus on the important aspects of your experience rather than side stories).

- Keep the focus and intention of the circle in mind when sharing.

Some of these qualities are life-long practices, so as facilitators we are inviting people to reflect consciously on their communication rather than expecting them to get these qualities right all the time.

Not offering solutions or aiming to fix situations or people

In everyday conversation, there can be a tendency to try to help people who share a difficult experience by offering solutions. However, this unsolicited advice can feel patronising, diminish the speaker's sense of being able to find their own solutions and/or shift the attention away from how the experience was towards an outcome.

We find repeatedly that when someone shares an experience, being properly listened to and having the feelings witnessed can bring incredible transformation, without any need to fix anything. Having this as a guideline can support attendees to feel that they can share something vulnerable without having then to sit through responses that may feel misguided or unhelpful.

Of course, someone in the circle can share a situation and explicitly ask for advice.

There are certain circumstances where facilitators or those with specific knowledge and experience can contribute. In these cases, it is recommended that the person who has spoken is asked if they would like to receive any guidance.

When Julia attended the Support after Murder and Manslaughter circle, she found many of the suggestions and experiences shared by seasoned facilitators and others in the group very helpful. In certain circumstances, signposting after someone has shared can be very useful, as can follow-up communication containing specific information.

Taking responsibility for yourself

Each individual has a duty to be self-aware in how they behave in the circle and to ask for support when needed (if they can). As a facilitator, you do not want someone to leave the circle and feel upset, unsupported and not wanting to return. It is not your job to provide hours of being a shoulder to cry on, but often a little support or signposting can diffuse the impact of a misunderstanding or the triggering of a past trauma. Tessa often jokes in her circles that she is unfortunately not psychic and so may not pick up on whether someone needs further support during a circle or afterwards.

If you know in advance that the circle will be emotive, more time can be spent on this guideline. For example, asking people to think about who they might talk to after the circle, tomorrow or in a week if things are stirred up is helpful. Reflecting on their support network and self-care often shows that they have resources in place.

The more emotive a topic, the more necessary it is to provide pauses and check-ins. You might repeat the settling practice from earlier and ask people to notice how their breathing is. Is it deep and calm or shallow and rapid? What emotions are here right now? What is needed to feel supported? It may also be appropriate for you to have organisations to which you can signpost attendees to access specialist support.

Taking responsibility for yourself also includes how people respond to others' feelings. If someone does get upset, does another attendee rush to get tissues to wipe tears away or give a hug? This may shut down someone's experience of expressing how they feel and signal that it's not okay to be upset. Gently communicating that all feelings are welcome and no feelings are too big or too much can support them to show up as they need to and signal for others to reflect on their own feelings first. You might need to reinforce this concept again and again.

It is your responsibility as circle holder to decide whether there needs to be another person or two responsible for the circle with you. When Julia attended a menopause circle where issues that could bring about distress were discussed, there was a trained menopause mentor present throughout who could support any person who needed to step out of the circle for additional support. In Daniel Groom's Queer Wellbeing circle, there would always be three facilitators present, each taking a different role so that additional support could be provided to individuals if required.

It is not always necessary to have more than one facilitator for a circle. However, taking responsibility for yourself includes the facilitator! Who would you turn to if you need support? In Chapter 10 we will be looking at what steps to take to care for yourself as a facilitator.

Timekeeping

Another aspect of the container of a circle is having a time boundary. You may decide that a circle is one hour, two hours or however long. Keeping to what you advertised, communicated or agreed is important as participants may have planned to be picked up from the circle, need to return to take over childcare or have other appointments or an early start in the morning. Describing what will happen and then sticking to that creates a feeling of safety and consistency over time.

Timekeeping is also key to the sharing process. The clearer the boundaries around the amount of time each person should speak for, the easier it can be to manage. This will relate to how many people attend the circle and how much time has been given for the length of the gathering. When there is a short amount of time, the response to a question posed in circle can be:

- one word

- three words

- a sentence

- a few sentences

- a minute

- two minutes.

Timekeeping is the responsibility of both the facilitator(s) and attendees of a circle. In most cases, a circle will have a clear start time when people are expected to have arrived and be ready for the opening. The facilitator needs to communicate this expectation clearly and reflect on what happens if someone is late. Having the contact details for people who have said they are attending means that you can check in with latecomers before starting the circle and potentially wait if they are running only slightly late.

If someone is habitually late, it is important to speak to them and find out if there is a reason. It might be that they use public transport and the bus times don't fit well with the start time. Perhaps another member of the circle can give them a lift. Perhaps there is an emotional or behavioural reason that you can help them reflect on. It can be important to share the impact of their coming late on how the circle runs as they might be unaware.

Alternatively, you might be in a setting like a festival where your intention is to give people a flavour of the circle process and allow people to join later. We suggest that you choose your topic carefully so that it doesn't matter if the container is not as strong as we normally would make it. (This is not to say that you cannot run a circle with a very strong container, but you would need to put clear expectations around arriving on time and staying in the circle where possible.)

Another reason that you might welcome latecomers is because your demographic has chaotic lives and it is enough of a challenge to get to the circle at all. In this situation, it would be useful to have a helper or co-facilitator so that there is someone who can welcome the person individually, explain where you are in the process of the circle and share the guidelines.

It is important to map your circle in terms of timing. Julia times her circles very tightly with 5–10-minute time-frame allocations. She also over-plans her circles so that there is potential for much to be covered and then tailors the length to ensure the circle does not run over the allotted time. This is often because there is a learning element to the circle and they often last two hours plus. However long your circle is, careful planning for timing is useful. Have clear aims and objectives for your circle. Write out your plan for the circle with time allocated for each section and make a note of what you will cut out if time runs away. Time as exactly as possible for each person to share. You can even practise with someone before the circle if you have a particular activity in mind to check how long a particular activity takes to complete.

It is important that you show clear authority with timekeeping. Participants relax when you hold timing well.

A responsibility of the facilitator is to finish the circle on time. In yoga ethics, we have the principle of 'asteya' or non-stealing; this relates not only to physical objects, but also to time. If you have communicated that the circle lasts two hours and then it continues for another hour, you have effectively stolen the other people's time. Perhaps they needed to leave for another appointment, to go to work, to go to bed to get up for work in the morning, for childcare reasons, because someone is waiting to give them a lift or they'll miss their bus.

Although you might ask people if they're okay with running over, this can put some people in an awkward position. They might not feel they can disrupt the circle by leaving, but it could massively inconvenience them. Others may feel comfortable with stating that they need to leave, miss out on the container being closed and feel the process is incomplete. Our suggestion, if you think that this may happen, is to communicate in advance that, for example, the circle will last for two hours and then there will be time afterwards for those who can stay to socialise. That way, you give the choice fairly to the attendees.

Time can magically disappear during a circle because we can become engrossed in listening to others. If you find timekeeping difficult, ask a participant who is good with timekeeping to give you a reminder 15 minutes before the circle is due to close or whenever you need to start the closing process. Explaining the timing of when different things will happen in the circle also provides a feeling of safety for all present. Ultimately, it is respectful to honour people's time.

When holding an in-person circle, it is important that you have easy access to a timepiece so you can literally keep an eye on the time. When Julia covered facilitation of a circle recently, she asked about the timepiece and ensured that she could see the clock. The circle she ran was in the middle of a fully scheduled day, so it was important that she started and finished at the expected time. If you are holding a circle in an unfamiliar space, it is important that you give yourself extra time to arrive and settle.

Now that you've heard about a range of possible guidelines, let's consider your personal experience of them and which are appropriate for your circle.

EXERCISE: REFLECTING ON VALUES

This exercise provides an opportunity to consider your experiences of these guidelines being shared and upheld well and not so well.

Think of the guidelines we have shared: confidentiality, respect, non-judgement, speaking from 'I' not 'you' or 'we', quality of speech, not giving solutions, taking responsibility for yourself and timekeeping.

Reflect on the times you have been in a space where these guidelines or others were used. How did it feel for that value to be upheld? What did it enable in you?

Now reflect on the situations where you were in a space where one or more of these values were not followed. How did it feel for you? What did you notice happened for other people? What happened next? Did you return to that space?

Take some time to reflect whether there are other guidelines that are appropriate to your circle. How would you express these values and why they are important to people who attend?

How can you practise sharing the guidelines if you are new to circle holding?

If you're already running circles, which guidelines are the most challenging for attendees to follow?

What is more appropriate for your circle: to share ready-made guidelines or co-create them?

This is how we might introduce the concept of the guidelines:

Before I open up the talking/introduce the topic, I want to remind you of the values we have for the circle. These are to create a place where people feel that they can share openly. I suggest the following guidelines: respect for each other (and different opinions); try to be non-judgemental and notice for yourself when judgement comes up; keep what is said in the circle confidential – it's fine for you to share your own experience but not other people's; talk about your own experience rather than what has happened to others; don't offer advice unless it's specifically requested;

and take responsibility for how you feel. If you need support at the end, please tell me as I might not realise otherwise. Thank you for arriving on time – I will finish on time in case you need to be off promptly.

You will find your own words for sharing guidelines. It might seem like a lot to cover, but it signals clearly how importantly you take the kind of communication that is going to happen at the gathering. You are setting the scene for reflective talking and respectful listening.

The concept of participation is included in the guidelines and pre-event invitation too, so that people know that their participation will be expected to be active rather than passive and that their involvement will be welcomed.

CIRCLE STORY: UPHOLDING BOUNDARIES
Mark Walsh specialises in embodiment circles. He shares:

> I have seen circles absolutely ruined by a lack of boundaries. I remember one I was in at the end of a movement event in Portugal. They just said, 'Right, we are going to share.' There were 30 people and they gave people as long as they wanted.

> Two hours later, I needed to pee. I was late to go to the thing I wanted to go to next. They had broken any kind of structure to it, and it got to my turn and I said I was bored and I want to go home. That's my shit and they got upset with me for saying I was bored. Sometimes the sharing isn't really allowed. Am bored, pissed off and I want to go home.

Mark found from experience that this tip works well:

> I use an electronic timer on my phone that beeps and it doesn't stop beeping. What that means is they don't take it personally when the timer goes off because they can see that it is fair for everyone. It is timed by a machine and it just keeps beeping. There are very few people who will continue speaking when there is a loud beeping noise. In AA they hold up a yellow card which is more gentle.

Timekeeping is an often overlooked, but important guideline. Here's an exercise to consider the issues around not keeping to time or setting healthy boundaries.

● EXERCISE: WHEN TIME GOES OUT THE WINDOW!

Read through this scenario and reflect on why this situation makes facilitation more challenging.

> Everyone arrived for the circle on time, got drinks and found a place to sit. The circle was marketed as two hours long. The facilitator opens the circle and invites people to introduce themselves with their name and whether they have come far. Then the guidelines are shared and people are invited to share if there is anything else they would like to add to the guidelines.
>
> Fifteen minutes into the circle, there's a knock at the door and three people have arrived who didn't book. The facilitator is a bit flustered but decides that they can join since they travelled 40 minutes to get to the venue. Space is made for the three latecomers by creating a bigger circle, and the facilitator feels it's important to go through the guidelines again. Still feeling stressed, the circle holder decides to give an impromptu settling practice to settle herself as much as the others.
>
> Thirty-five minutes pass before the topic is introduced. It's a lively group and there is lots of sharing of experiences. The time goes quickly, and the facilitator realises that it is already five minutes past the closing time. She announces that the end of the circle has come already and asks people to share one word that sums up how they are feeling to close the gathering.
>
> One person says that they're really enjoying the circle and it seems a shame to stop, looking around for agreement from others. Someone else shares that there's something they'd really like to express before leaving, and so it continues. A couple of people are fidgeting and looking at their watch. In the end, they get up to go and find out later that the circle had continued for another 90 minutes.

What issues did you notice while reading the scenario? Is there anything that the facilitator could have done to prevent or remedy these issues? What learning points feel important for how you would hold a circle?

There is a lot to consider in this chapter. Please don't feel overwhelmed, but know that in time you will find your authentic way of framing the circle. Not all of the guidelines will be relevant for your circle, but providing some kind of structure for communication will enhance the experience for everyone.

It's hard to 100 per cent guarantee that setting up guidelines for the circle will mean that everyone will feel safe all the time, but by reflecting on what a brave space means, we can work towards talking respectfully even when there might be different views or uncertainty about how to talk about certain subjects. We need to be aware that the spaces we hold may not be suitable for everyone, and that is okay. One of the purposes of this book is to provide the tools for anyone who wishes to create a circle, to benefit a demographic you care about.

In the next chapter, we suggest different ways of introducing a topic for your circle and how to plan your time.

CHAPTER 9

Topics, Themes, Planning and Scheduling

The feeling of a container has been built through the introductions, settling and sharing of guidelines. You can see that some people are eager to express themselves and perhaps you ask, 'What is happening for you today?' and let the talking unfold. Or perhaps you have an idea of something to lead to a deeper level of sharing. Creating a theme for your circle creates a wonderful sense of continuity from beginning to end.

When you first thought of facilitating a circle, you may have started with the question 'What shall we talk about?' Start by identifying 'Who is this circle for and what do they need?' In addressing their needs, you will decide how to guide the talking in the circle. You might decide that one of these approaches would be most appropriate:

- a general invitation to share

- A topic related to the reason for meeting (e.g. consent in a teen wellbeing circle)

- A theme for the whole event (e.g. celebrating the summer solstice).

A general invitation to share

It might be that the reason for holding a circle is to create a space to share whatever is uppermost in people's minds on the day. Reflective questions such as the following can open the talking:

- What is alive for you right now?

- What do you want to voice?

- What stands out in your experiences over the last month? (If it's a monthly circle.)

- When you pause, what is coming up for you?

- What has brought you here today?

Be aware that asking such open-ended questions can lead to long responses, so it's important to give an indication of the amount of time someone should speak for, whether it's three words, one or two sentences or two minutes, if you want to enable everyone to have an opportunity to speak. Providing a container with these questions makes facilitation easier and enables everyone in the circle to have a chance to speak.

We don't use 'How are you today?' because people may launch into a big description of everything that is happening in their life. More reflective questions like the ones above will provide a different kind of answer. Asking 'How are you today?' can also make someone wonder, 'Where do I start? There's so much going on,' and freeze up.

This type of checking in can be so valuable for all types of groups and acts as a safety valve for those who don't have any other space to be heard about their experiences of life. Often themes will emerge naturally as people respond to each other with shared experiences or different experiences of the same situation. This can be a person-centred way of working that gives control over what to speak about to those attending rather than pre-deciding a topic.

Not having a topic to introduce can create more time for sharing. While there is incredible value in being witnessed in your current experience, the risk is that the talking jumps from experience to experience and, without careful facilitation, an uncovering of deeper personal understanding doesn't happen.

Another aspect to consider is whether you are hoping there will be regular attendees at a repeating circle or even a closed group of participants. The possibility to have a deeper level of sharing is usually easier as circle attendees become familiar with each other. A shared understanding arises of what the aim of the circle time is, from the commitment of showing up regularly and witnessing one another over time.

Tessa shares:

One lady came for years to my Red Tent circle and was for many months very introverted. The circle met on the Monday nearest the new moon and this was when she had her period. After a year, though, her cycle shifted and she attended the gathering when she was nearing ovulation. It was like having a different person at the event. She was humorous and playful. It was a great lesson in remembering that we see a snapshot of someone at a talking circle. We laughed about it later.

If you are using circle time as a small element of something else, like a yoga class or workshop, questions like the following might be most helpful:

- How was that practice experienced by you?

- How are you feeling about the information at this point in the workshop?

- How is the information landing?

- Thinking about what we've done so far, how do you feel in your body?

Alternatively, it might be that you will have different participants each time because it's a drop-in circle, in a temporary setting like a festival or created as a one-off experience. A Narrative 4 'story exchange' is used as the form for their circles, which is a type of mirroring activity, purposively bringing people together from different backgrounds to connection. Lee Keylock explains:

> When two people in our method come together, you are sharing a story from your life, any story. It could be funny, sad, embarrassing. You can keep it all positive at first if you would like to. The idea is that you give them space for 20 minutes each. You model the types of stories people tell: just everyday stories. The idea is to be present when the other person is talking. You then narrate the story back in the first person. You take your partner's story, and they take yours. You tell their story back in the first person as if it is your own.

> [In the big circle], your partner is sitting there. You are not telling your own story in the circle. Telling the story as if it is your own really collapses the distance between people. It is very hard to dismiss a person or see them as a caricature or stereotype once you know something personal about them. You fully embody the life of someone else for a minute. It gets you closer to someone else's experience. It frees you up to be present.

You might wish to create a specific formula like this for your circle that is unique. When hosting a circle with people who don't know each other, whether it's because it's the first ever circle or a one-off event, having a structure in place to support them through the experience is key.

Regular talking circles

In a regular talking circle, the same questions might be used as prompts every time you meet. These questions may relate to the reason for meeting, such as menstrual cycle awareness (see the example below). In a grief circle, providing a topic is often not necessary, especially if the participants in the group are different each week. The regular question asked in a grief circle might be 'How has your week been?' Obviously, the container needs to be well held for this type of circle. It is a chance for attendees to talk about their lived experience around a common issue.

Example: Suggested questions for a regular circle on menstrual cycles

With short circles of 60 minutes or less, there does not need to be a specific topic. For example, a menstrual cycle circle with 8–12 girls talking about their menstrual cycle in the school lunch break can have the same questions each week.

- What day of your cycle are you on?

- What season of your cycle do you feel you are in?

- What is coming up for you?

Clarification about the menstrual cycle may be needed for new joiners. A topic may naturally emerge from the girls' experiences, but there does not need to be anything additional to this sharing of experiences.

Remember that it is helpful for the facilitator to begin speaking, because you model the level of sharing (e.g. intensity of experience, length of talking). For example, when Julia runs her menopause workshops, once short introductions have been made and the event has been framed, she will talk from her own perspective about her experience of perimenopause. Once she has shared her experience, she then invites others to share.

Providing a topic in a regular circle can extend attendees' reflections on their experience and bring variety to the gathering. A topic can also add to the psychological container that supports people to share their experiences. For example, you might hold a circle for new parents with different topics each week. Having a topic of 'sex after birth' or 'mothers' mental load' gives people a feeling of permission to talk about taboo or sensitive topics that they might not normally bring up.

Another example is that you might have a circle that meets monthly to talk about concerns for the local environment. Topics that you might introduce from month to month could be how to support children who are worried about the environment, small actions that can be taken in everyday life or creating a community day to raise awareness. You can ask the circle participants what concerns they have or listen out for issues while people are chatting over tea.

You may have an idea to create a circle because you specifically wish to look at issues that face your community. This is something that Daniel Groom felt was needed to build support within the LGBTQIA+ community and common understanding between different generations who had experienced different challenges. He shares the responsibility for the circle with two colleagues who come from different parts of the LGBTQIA+ community, so between them they can discuss which topics to introduce and how best to introduce them to the group.

CIRCLE STORY: MAKING SENSE OF LIFE'S CHALLENGES

Julia shares:

> When I was a teenager, I ran a weekly Jewish youth group with local friends. Each week we created space to discuss in circle an issue that we were facing. We were brought up to address one of the most difficult historical topics: the Holocaust. We grappled with questions about how a community could be betrayed, what it means to take a stand for someone else when your own life and that of your family would be at risk, how to live our lives as Jewish teenagers within a community where we were experiencing anti-Semitism, with friends who attended Jewish schools experiencing physical and verbal abuse on the way to school and security guards required at the gates because of threats of violence to the community.
>
> How could we as teenagers learn more about Middle Eastern politics,

because we were expected to both understand and have views due to our religion. We would soften the challenges of talking about these issues in circle with singing together and creating opportunities to have fun too!

The group I was part of was for 14–17-year-olds and I only remember adults being involved as educators when we went on summer and winter camping holidays. So the themes of our circle came directly from our needs as Jewish teenagers growing up in multicultural London where teenagers from other cultures were also learning how to rub alongside us. I have always greatly valued living in the melting pot that is London while having the security of my teenage Jewish circle to talk about the tricky aspects of life which were specific to my difference.

What you care about and the specific needs of the community you serve will shape the questions and topics that are introduced in your circle. The next exercise will help you to get the talking off to a good start in a regular circle. We will look at one-off events later in the chapter.

● EXERCISE: WHAT DO PEOPLE WANT AND NEED TO TALK ABOUT?

Have paper and a pen to hand to write down or draw your responses. Think about the people who will attend your circle and the experiences they will want to talk about. Decide whether you are planning this to be a regular circle or a one-off event.

- Do you want to keep it simple and ask people to share their current experience? Write three or four reflective questions you can use.

- Are there regular questions that will be relevant at every circle you facilitate because of your shared characteristics or shared interest? List a few.

- Will a different topic each time be supportive of widening people's reflections on their experience? Knowing the demographic, write down five issues that concern them.

- If you're finding it difficult to come up with issues, where can you find ideas? (e.g. socially, in a relevant Facebook group, on an Instagram account of someone in the demographic that you follow)

Once you know what your regular questions or topics are going to be, sharing a relevant reading is a wonderful way to set the scene.

Sharing a relevant reading

We often start with a poem, story or reading that speaks to the topic. This can set the tone for the talking and enable people to enter a more reflective space. As they listen, they can think how what the author conveys relates to their own experience. Give time for the words to be absorbed before expecting people to respond or without any expectation of a response. Allowing silence supports those in the circle to have time to gather their thoughts and think about what to share if you are asking for how the reading has landed. However, there is no need for them to respond to what you have shared. It is enough that they have heard the words and that maybe something has resonated.

Once you have shared a reading, it is a good time to give people the space and time to share their reason for being in the circle. If you have introduced a topic to a group of regular circle attendees, you can ask something like:

- How does the reading [poem/story] resonate with your own experience?

- How did those words make you feel?

- Can you relate to what the author shared?

Let people have a chance to think about your question before expecting a response. If it seems as if people don't know where to start, you could share your own reaction or why you chose the piece.

Recently, Julia shared a poem about gratitude in her yoga circle. Some of the people listening to the poem talked about aspects of it that resonated with them, and the circle grew into talking about what each of us felt grateful for and how gratitude can positively impact our lives. The topic that grew out of the poem was gratitude in the face of adversity.

Other general topics that Julia regularly uses in her yoga circles are exhaustion; rest; rule breaking; anger; sadness; joy; the difference between aggression, assertiveness and passivity; the wonder of the physical body and its functionality in juxtaposition to the way it looks; and menstruation. These topics reflect that Julia is working within the realm of yoga and all of these themes can be looked at both somatically through physical practice and through the mechanism of the talking circle.

Sharing information

Another way to introduce a topic is to provide some information so that everyone has a similar level of knowledge to share from. For example, if you are running a circle about perimenopause, you might need to give definitions for perimenopause, menopause and post-menopause. If menstrual cycle awareness is your topic, explaining what Day 1 means in relation to the cycle, and terms like luteal and follicular, would help those who know less to be included in the sharing. Perhaps you're holding a circle for carers and you explain that you're focusing on the carer finding space for themselves rather than sharing about the person they care for. You could give an example of carers' needs by showing them some hard-hitting statistics about the mental health of carers as a discussion opener.

We see the difference between a talking circle and a workshop in the amount of teaching that happens. In a talking circle, the teaching of a subject is minimal. In a workshop, more time is given to teaching, with a small proportion of the time used for sharing how the information and practices have been experienced. In a pure talking and listening circle, there would not be any teaching from one person. We can learn from everyone's life experiences and they're all held as equally valid and important.

Exploring through journalling

If the topic is sensitive, emotional, philosophical or taboo, journalling can provide a stepping stone to talking about it. Providing several questions and inviting people to write their responses as a stream of consciousness is helpful. For this, you would need to communicate before the event to bring paper and a pen or have sufficient to provide for everyone. Also give the option for people to draw or doodle if that suits them better. Make it clear at the start that people won't need to share everything they write or draw, as otherwise they might hold back on what they express on paper.

People will vary in how long they will write for. Watch for when half the people have finished and give a couple more minutes for the others to finish their sentence. Invite them to return to the journalling after the circle if they have more to write.

Then invite people to share what came up for them during the journalling. They can choose which parts they feel comfortable to share and which parts will remain private.

Using icebreakers to introduce a topic

A way to get a discussion of a tricky topic going is to ask people to write down their hopes and fears around the topic on post-it notes, collect them in, shuffle them and read them out anonymously. Another way is to get them to rate their stress levels about talking on the topic between 1 and 10 so you can gauge the vibe in the room (no explanation is needed about why they feel that level). Once you reconfirm confidentiality, they may be more confident speaking when they realise others are feeling nervous.

If you choose a topic that could bring about strong emotions, you may wish to give people guidelines about how they respond. A sliding scale can be helpful for this – for example, 'If you are thinking of sharing, with 1 being the least emotive and 10 the most, you might wish to start with a 4–5.' This can be helpful to avoid 'vulnerability hangovers' as Brene Brown calls that feeling of having shared too much, after the event. However, due to the very nature of the topic in some circles, most of the sharing could be at the top of the range.

To give you an example, one of Tessa's trainees wanted to start an online circle for mums who were immigrants to the UK, being one herself. For her first circle, she chose the topic of 'Mothering through the pandemic'. She reflected afterwards that this was a challenging subject because the mums were either still feeling incredibly emotional about the experience or had blocked it out in the busyness of everyday life. Big, raw emotions contrasted with others not knowing what to say and feelings of numbness. Talking with a couple of people who match your demographic before the circle can help you gauge how the topic might land.

Rather than going round the circle in order, you can invite people to take the talking stick (see the section 'Creating the right atmosphere' in Chapter 5) and speak when they feel ready. This allows people who are ready to speak to start sharing their experiences while others decide whether they want to talk or listen. Before the next person speaks, it can be helpful for the facilitator to say, 'Thank you for sharing,' or ask everyone to join in with that or something similar to acknowledge the person who has spoken. This creates a pause to differentiate from everyday conversation where speech bounces backwards and forwards.

Revisiting your intention for the circle will support your choice of topic (see the exercise 'Intention setting' in Chapter 3). What is most relevant to the people who you are hoping will attend? Whether the attendees are new to the circle experience or are regulars may also be a factor in the topic you choose. If attendees are new, you might choose a subject that is less challenging to talk about. A new circle is like a new friendship.

Here is a specific example of a quarterly circle for mothers and daughters who wanted to focus on preparing for puberty. There is a different topic for each circle that is relevant to the participants' needs. Your circles' attendees and their needs may be very different, but hopefully this provides an example from which you can imagine fleshing out a topic for your demographic. If you are interested in using complementary activities like crafts or running circles with children, you will find more detail in Chapters 13 and 14.

Example: Mother and daughter circles

The following is based on the series of four in-person circles run with co-facilitator Catherine Holt. The girls were 7–9 years old.

Circle 1: Cycles and emotions

- Opening: Name, and what's your favourite season?

- Circle guidelines

- Activity: Colouring mandalas related to inner seasons

- Initial round: What life cycles can you think of? (Frogs, butterflies, people, etc.)

- Topic questions: What big emotions do you have sometimes? (Using cards with pictures that describe emotions, such as Bear cards – see Resources)

- Does Mummy's emotions change over the month? If so, how?

- What can we do with big emotions?

- Closing: Pick a strength card for your mum/daughter

Circle 2: Changing bodies

- Opening: Name, and what animal would you be and why?

- Circle guidelines

- Activity: Drawing and colouring a uterus angel (see Figure 9.1)

- Initial round: How does your body change as you get older?

- Teaching: Use a uterus apron (an apron with a diagram of a uterus on the front that is positioned over that part of the anatomy) to talk about internal anatomy

- Topic questions (to mums): What do you remember from puberty? (Emailed beforehand so they could think about useful experiences to share)

- Closing (to girls): How do you feel about the things you've heard today? (Bear emotion cards)

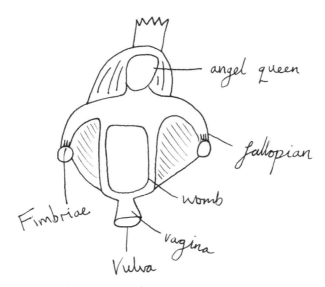

Figure 9.1 'Angel uterus' created by Henrietta

Circle 3: Periods

- Opening: Name, and what's your favourite way of feeling snuggly/cosy?

- Circle guidelines

- Activity: Making collage cards

- Initial round: How old was your mum when she had her first period?

- Teaching: Showing range of period products

- Topic questions: What do you know about periods? How can you look after yourself the whole month?

- Activity: Writing a message for your future self in the card you made

- Closing: How could you help your mum next time she has her period?

Circle 4: Celebrating the feminine

- Opening: Name, and can you think of a woman who has a super-power, like music, writing, running, dancing or something else?

- Circle guidelines

- Activity: Making clay goddesses (or something else you want to make)

- Topic questions (mums): Which woman has had a big impact in your life? (Emailed beforehand so they could think about some-one to talk about and possibly bring a photo/significant object)

- Teaching: Big emotions and how we look after ourselves as we change/through the month

- Activity: Fire ceremony – explain letting go of things, ask the participants to write down on paper things they would like to let go of, and put the paper into a fire (optional) with lavender and rosemary

- Closing: Short sound bath snuggling with Mum. (A sound bath is a relaxation practice where you 'bathe' in the vibrations of sound made by a gong, singing bowls and other instruments.)

The opening in these circles uses a simple or fun question as an icebreaker. The initial activities in these gatherings were used as a settling practice that continues while talking about these topics. Rather than the facilitators teaching too much, asking the mums to share while the girls are busy with craft activities means they hear a range of experiences.

● EXERCISE: CIRCLE TIME ON HOLIDAY, AT WORKSHOPS, FESTIVALS AND RETREATS

If you are thinking about creating a circle and are not sure where to start, try this exercise. You might be going on holiday or doing an activity with family or friends and could try out this simple circle holding practice. It can easily be adapted for use at festivals and at the end of workshops and retreats.

> Julia goes on an annual holiday with her extended family. It has become a tradition at the end of every day when gathering around the dinner table together for the question to be asked of each person: 'What is your highlight of the day?'
>
> It is likely that a highlight will involve another family member, and a sense of community is built together with a combined sense of satisfaction because of the accumulated happy memories. Often there is some humour in the stories told and they are likely to reveal something of the character of the person sharing. It will also give everyone an opportunity to hear about the range of activities that have taken place that day. However the day may have turned out, everyone always manages to find a highlight to talk about.
>
> There are norms that have been simply created around this tradition. Everyone has to be seated at the table before the sharing begins. Each person speaks without being interrupted by someone else. Anyone can start by asking the question and each person speaks in turn around the table to ensure every person is heard. As this tradition takes place each night of the holiday, the question is usually introduced by a different person each night and the order of speaking also changes. It is an opportunity for a family community with ages ranging from pre-teens to seventies to listen to each other.
>
> There is value in asking this question when you are running a larger event because it provides feedback you can use. If a number of people have experienced the same highlight, that could affect the choices you make when you run an event in future. You might find the choices people make surprising.

In Chapter 11, we will look in more detail at reflective questions you can use to close a circle.

Talking and listening circles are fantastic for allowing difficult subjects to be addressed, and we would love you to be courageous in your intentions for your circle holding. The basic structure can be used for a whole spectrum of intentions, from sharing holiday highlights to addressing taboo subjects to supporting conflict resolution.

For example, Narrative 4 uses their story exchange in relation to a 'Guns and Empathy' project, and they also bring Arabs and Israelis together for story sharing and talking circles: 'The shortest distance between two people is a story' (Lee Keylock).

Creating a theme for one-off events

What if you want to create a theme for a circle from beginning to end? We differentiate between a topic and a theme to illustrate that you might have a different topic for a circle, and everything else (opening, settling practice, closing) stays very similar for a regular event, whereas with a theme everything is chosen to relate back to it.

Imagine a wedding for a moment. The event is all about the happy couple who have chosen music that they love and a venue that suits their personalities and background (traditional religious service or yurt in a field?); perhaps they have photos of themselves as youngsters at the reception and wedding favours that hint at their style or hobbies or sense of humour. Everything is themed around a common focus.

It can be similar for a circle.

Perhaps you want to mark a particular time of the year like a solstice or Christmas. Sacred times in the year are a natural time for people to gather and can provide the opportunity for celebration. Of course, you could hold a quarterly circle whose aim is to mark the winter solstice, spring equinox, summer solstice and autumn equinox. Julia likes to run yoga nidra events on these dates.

Or maybe you want to hold a longer event like a day retreat or a residential retreat over a few days. Having a theme supports your creation of content so that it holds together and there is a feeling of consistency. This is all part of creating a container for sole or group work.

Just as you thought about your intention for holding a circle for a particular demographic to meet their needs, reflect on what your aim is for creating this circle. Perhaps you want to give people deep rest away from the everyday world and so you have a theme of rest and rejuvenation. The reading you might share, the settling practices, the questions to start off the talking could all be based on rest and rejuvenation. If you have refreshments or a lunch included, you might include drinks and foods that support the theme.

Here is a specific example of the theme of spring equinox for a one-off event. You might not be interested in marking the spring equinox, but hopefully you can use this as an example of how to include the theme in the choices you make for different components of the circle.

Example: Spring equinox circle theme

Set-up: Mandala created out of spring flowers for a centrepiece

People invited to bring an object that symbolises spring and new life (add around centrepiece)

Opening: Name, and how does it feel to be in spring for you? (two words each)

Settling practice: Visualisation – imagine yourself as a dormant tree in winter, then moving into spring with sap rising and leaves ready to unfurl. What wants to express itself as that happens?

Topic: Share words from Glennie Kindred's *The Earth's Cycle of Celebration*

Journalling prompts – What plans have been incubating over winter?

What new activity will you give energy to?

What do you wish to bring out into the world?

How will you look after yourself as you manifest?

Listening partnership (see Chapter 10): Share what came up with the other person

Teaching: Alder tree sits at the spring equinox in the Wheel of the Year – known for underlying energy, taking up challenges, facing hidden things (from Glennie Kindred's *The Sacred Tree*). Have a branch to show and catkins to pass around.

Circle question: What have you discovered from your reflections so far?

Celebration: Sharing of poems, songs, music (emailed before so people can prepare something – optional)

Closing: Share one word for how you feel at the close of the circle

Gift of seeds

Suzan Nolan, of Gather the Women, talks about how starting with one theme led her to long-term participation in circles on the international political stage:

> In the early 80s someone said to me, 'Would you like to be in a circle about feminine spirituality?' I had no idea what this meant, none, I just said yes because I knew this woman... We have had circles in the United Nations when we went to the Commission on the status of women and in the Parliament of World Religions.

Talking and listening circles can be on a small scale in someone's living room to mark a personal occasion or take place on an international level.

Weaving a theme through a circle can take time to prepare but is also a lot of fun. The next exercise supports you in this process.

● EXERCISE: BURST OPEN YOUR CREATIVITY

Read through this exercise and then draw, write or speak aloud about what comes up.

Think about your intention for the circle and imagine the people who will attend. Without judging what you're writing, write down as many words that you can think of related to your intention, the shared interest or characteristics of those that will come.

Now pick out a word and write down all the associated ideas you have with it. For example, when I chose 'vulnerability', I came up with Brene Brown, child, tender, weakness, strength, shield, scared, the song 'Kind' by Copper Wimmin.

Which of the words will help people understand what the circle event is about? Can you turn it into a positive theme? For example, from vulnerability to 'finding your greatest strength in vulnerability'.

You could go to the internet and search for a poem about your keywords, look for a reading for any authors or songs that you thought of, or write down a definition of the word.

Does the theme lend itself to something visual for a centrepiece or decoration of the venue? For example, for finding strength in vulnerability I would look for natural items that looked fragile but were actually strong, or a symbol of transformation like a butterfly's cocoon.

Do any of the associated words give you an idea about an initial question that could be used in a check-in round that introduces the topic gently?

Could you use any of the words in a settling practice so that you're building connections to what you'll talk about later?

What open-ended questions could you use to ask about the theme?

Take a breath and step back from the detail. What feels most important about theme? Come back in a few days and add to your ideas.

Breaking down the event into smaller activities will help you get started if you feel overwhelmed. You will find your own way to plan a themed event.

> I planned the circles by staring into space and imagining, writing notes by hand and typing on the laptop. I needed to dig deep to excavate the topics my heart wanted to share...topics such as embodiment, masculine and feminine, a feminine way of being, real sensual relationship, appreciation for the earth, and more. I read a lot, and brought aspects of workshops, retreats and professional trainings I'd attended. Often, I created new meditations and exercises for the participants to enjoy and learn from.
>
> *Julia Paulette Hollenbery*

Creating a schedule for your circle

Now that we've considered what the main part of the talking and listening circle may look like, let's think about how much time we spend on different parts of the gathering. Obviously, this is going to be different depending on how long the circle is. Here are templates for 45-minute, one-hour and two-hour circles. These are rough guides to get you started.

Example: 45-minute circle schedule (for up to ten people)

Let's assume this is an online circle and you have invited people to come into the meeting room five minutes before the start time. You can have a waiting room set up on Zoom so people know you are there and then open exactly on time or admit people as they arrive and chat. We are also assuming there are ten people in this circle.

0–2 mins   Welcome, request to have videos on

3–5 mins	Explanation of guidelines
6–10 mins	Initial check-in of two words each
11–15 mins	Settling practice with eyes closed or looking away from screen
16–20 mins	Reading/poem and introduction of topic
20–25 mins	Opening question and sharing of own experience on the topic
25–40 mins	Talking and listening
40–45 mins	Closing check-out

Example: One-hour circle schedule (for up to 12 people)

(Before start) Arrival and welcoming

0–10 mins	Initial check-in – once round the circle in order
11–15 mins	Short settling practice
16–20 mins	Poem and reflection time, reminder of guidelines
21–50 mins	Topic introduced (if applicable), questions to start talking and invitation to talk if anyone feels the impulse to
51–58 mins	Closing check-in – round the circle in order
59–60 mins	Closing gesture (e.g. smiling to everyone in the room) and reminder of date of next circle
(after circle)	Social time for half an hour

Example: Two-hour circle schedule (8–10 participants)

(15 mins before start) Arrival and welcoming

0–10 mins	Welcome with names, where you have travelled from and what brought you here – give guidelines of 3–4 sentences

10–15 mins	Group guidelines and outline for the session
15–25 mins	Short settling practice with simple breathwork followed by a short reading (see Chapter 7)
25–35 mins	Short embodiment practice with movement (see Chapter 7)
35–50 mins	Explanation of listening partnerships and five-minute practice in pairs related to the needs of the group demographic (see Chapter 10 for listening partnerships)
50–70 mins	Discussion of the listening partnership experience speaking from own experience
70–80 mins	Short rest break with shared food – e.g. a piece of chocolate/dried fruit
80–100 mins	Expanded story share from each person related to theme for session (ten people would allow for two minutes each)
100–105	Short embodiment practice
105–110	Create frame for next gathering with themes
110–120	One-sentence takeaway

(Allow for 15 mins after the event for leave-taking)

The shorter the circle, the tighter the facilitator needs to be with timing. For short gatherings, give clear boundaries, such as using one- or two-word check-ins and timing people's sharing for two or five minutes if there are lots of people.

With longer gatherings, we like to over-plan with more content than is needed and a very tight time structure. That allows for you as a facilitator to relax a little, knowing that there are sufficient activities to fill the time, but you will also need to be flexible and leave things out if you have given additional space for a specific aspect of the circle.

The more confident you become with the topics of your circle, the less you will need to prepare in advance. It is really important that you create your timing schedule around the number of people in attendance so you are clear about how much time to allow for sharing for each person if you are looking to give everyone an equal opportunity to speak.

Creating topics and themes can be one of the most satisfying parts of holding circles because you can broaden people's reflections about their lives and a special, even sacred, atmosphere can be produced. A topic or theme can be part of the container that is created by the facilitator(s), and part of the magic, so that the sharing flows and the people attending discover something new about themselves. Even when a topic is challenging, as in a grief circle, a short event can work well if you keep tight boundaries. When you as the circle holder have a clear intention for the circle, the people who attend will be more likely to have clarity too.

In the next chapter, we address circle dynamics so that you can feel more confident managing the talking and keeping to your timings.

CHAPTER 10

Circle Dynamics

You're noticing that the same people keep taking up the thread of the topic in the circle today. You wonder if those that have been quiet haven't found a chance to share or are content with listening. When you check in with them, they decide to speak, and you realise how closely they've been listening to the sharing. The dynamic shifts and a new thread emerges.

A container is created for the circle by sharing guidelines and explicitly explaining the etiquette for the gathering. This supports people to understand what the expectations are around communication and can be a welcome relief when so much of interaction in normal life follows unwritten rules. However, despite this process of framing how to be together, people in the circle will have different amounts to say, and there may be disagreements or feelings of discomfort, or other dynamics at play. This chapter is about how to manage circle dynamics.

Depth of sharing

One issue that came up when interviewing people about their experience of holding circles was knowing how deep to take the talking. One person thought that facilitators might misjudge how deep or private an experience someone is willing to share. The key is not to have expectations of what experiences will be shared, and then we can meet someone exactly where they are. This is where the framing is important: if you've laid the groundwork for all emotions being welcome, of people not rushing in to fix the problem or wipe up tears, and have mechanisms for containing these bigger sharings, it will be okay!

If you suspect that a topic is going to bring up a lot of emotion and pain, it is important to start the circle with an invitation to share something lighter or set a container of time for each person. Sharing a settling practice at the beginning that can be returned to or asking people what inner resources they have to comfort themselves can also be helpful.

For example, in peri-/menopause circles very difficult emotional and physical symptoms and rage can come up quickly. It's important to pace the circle and not scare people who are not used to circling or weren't expecting that level of sharing. For example, you can set a time for two minutes of sharing for the first round. This signals that we are dipping our toe into what is present, letting people settle and hearing everyone's voices before a round of deeper sharing.

It could be helpful to give people a guideline of the depth of sharing. You might say, 'When you share, if you imagine a scale from 1 to 10 with 1 being the lightest and 10 being the most emotionally charged, I recommend you start by sharing a 3–4 rather than going straight to your 10.' Doing this in initial rounds supports people who tend to overshare to hear from others and get a sense of the level of sharing before deciding whether to share something bigger later.

You can also use this tool the other way around if you find people are undersharing and staying in everyday chat mode. First, reflect on the container you have created. Did you spend enough time settling people and going through the guidelines for respectful communication? You could say, 'When you share, if you imagine a scale from 1 to 10 with 1 being the lightest and 10 being the most emotionally charged, it seems that we are at 1. I wonder what would support you to move to a 3–4?' If as the facilitator you can share something at level 3–4, that will model what level of reflective sharing you're hoping to encourage.

If someone is dominating the talking

Sometimes it will be appropriate to interject when a person is talking at length and dominating the circle time. As the facilitator, when the person pauses for breath, you could say, 'Let's just pause for a moment at this point in the circle. That's a lot you've just spoken about. Shall we hear from the others about their experience of [e.g. overwhelm, isolation]?' You can clarify that you're not looking for feedback, solutions or responses to what the person has shared, but other people's experience on the topic. In this way, you're not in danger of dismissing the person's experience by moving on to something completely different but providing an opportunity for others to speak.

If the person has moved into telling a big story including others' actions and feelings, remind them gently to talk from 'I' about their experience today of the situation. Perhaps they can express how they feel in the present, their felt sense, rather than narrating the twists and turns of the whole story. Taking a break and asking someone else to put the kettle on and getting a fresh round of drinks can give you an opportunity to check in with the talker.

> A lot of women who came [to my early circles] had no awareness of how to share. Sometimes they would come along once, share their trauma and never come again. Sometimes, the Red Tent and the Goddess Circles went on a journey I wasn't prepared to go on. I had to bring in suggestions with regard to sharing time.
>
> *Lisa Horwell*

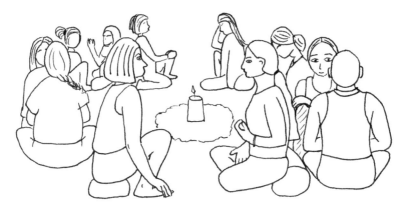

Figure 10.1 Listening partnerships within a circle

Having a topic to direct the talking can help prevent someone getting a traumatic experience off their chest at the expense of others having an opportunity to speak. If someone is recounting a very challenging experience, it *is* hard to interrupt them, but if the circle has a topic as part of the container rather than an open invitation to share what is present, this can support a gradual opening up. It also allows a facilitator to draw people back to the focus of the circle.

Another useful tool for ensuring that everyone has a chance to speak is listening partnerships. In the exercise below you will be shown how they work and also be given tips for introducing them into your circle. They can be used in person and also online in breakout rooms (a breakout room for each pair).

● EXERCISE: HOW TO USE LISTENING PARTNERSHIPS

If you are going to use listening partnerships in your circle, it's important that you have experienced them yourself. Find a willing person to practise with.

The concept is simple. The purpose of a listening partnership is to practise speaking without interruption and listening without comment. Julia was introduced to the concept of listening partnerships by a friend who also had very young children. They found each other through the organisation Hand in Hand Parenting (www.handinhandparenting.org).

Round 1

Person 1 – The Speaker: Speaks for five minutes without interruption. It's helpful to give a question for the person to respond to or a topic to talk around. For example:

> 'What's your experience of [grief, menstrual cycle awareness, being a new parent etc]?'

> 'What are the barriers and positive steps to moving forwards?'

> 'What is alive for you today?' (Although this is a big question, you make it clear there is a set time to talk.)

Person 2 – The Listener: The listener can show that they are listening by nodding, making eye contact, making suitable facial expressions and making sounds of following like 'Mmm', but they are not to speak. This can be difficult and may even feel rude if you are used to showing that you are listening by saying things like 'Oh yes, I understand,' 'I know exactly what you mean,' or 'I had that same experience.' It is important to keep within the guidelines and remain silent however strong the urge is to speak.

It is the responsibility of the listener to keep time.

Clearing questions

At the end of five minutes, the listener asks clearing questions: these are questions that are totally unrelated to the topic that the person has been speaking about. The questions need to be basic.

Examples are:

> 'When you look around you, what are the first three objects that you see?'

> 'What did you eat at your last meal?'

'What are you wearing on your feet?'

'What is your favourite flower?'

A recommended number of clearing questions would be three. They should be closed questions: questions that can be answered directly with a very few words.

Round 2
Once the clearing questions have been asked, the roles are reversed and the other person speaks for the same length of time.

Rejoining the circle
Once people have finished, invite them to share their experience. Remind them to talk from 'I'. They can share their own experience of hearing the other person talk but not the content. They are welcome to share their own content of what they talked about and the experience of being listened to. If they found the practice helpful, you can invite them to arrange to continue the partnership outside of the circle.

The exercise may be challenging for the speaker if they are used to others interjecting when talking. It is fine if there is silence if the speaker is thinking about what to say next or has run out of things to say. Listening partnerships are about practising the art of listening and witnessing someone's experience.

We have found that starting listening partnerships with five minutes each builds confidence. Even in this very short space of time, the benefits of speaking without interruption and listening without responding can be felt. In longer circles, you can include multiple listening partnerships either with the same partners or different partners. As confidence grows, you can also introduce longer sharing times.

If you create a regular listening partnership, it is helpful to agree a consistent time that you will talk each week or each month. Our advice is to keep to the time you have agreed in advance and keep chatting to another occasion. You can meet in person, over the phone or via a platform like Zoom.

When you are ready to introduce listening partnerships into your circle, practise explaining how it works. Check if people have questions and everyone has a partner. If there is an odd number of people, you can either have a triad or be in a pair yourself. Allow extra time for changing over and the interactions that inevitably happen afterwards. For five minutes each sharing, we suggest allowing at least 15 minutes for the activity.

Supporting roles

We'll talk about co-facilitation later in the book, but something that can be helpful is to have people with supporting roles for the circle gathering. If timekeeping is your weakness, appointing someone to be a timekeeper who can let you know when the circle is halfway through and 15 minutes before the end would be helpful.

Depending on the nature of the circle, you might also appoint someone to welcome latecomers or be available for anyone who has become upset and wants time outside the circle to be accompanied. It might also be appropriate to invite someone to have the role of the guardian, as explained by Suzan Nolan of Gather the Women (GTW):

> The role of the guardian comes from Christina Baldwin and Ann Linnea who wrote the book *The Circle Way*. Because it is hard for a circle leader or circle tender to catch all the dynamics of a circle, the guardian is the person who watches the sometimes very nuanced changes in the circle energy.

> We say that everyone in the circle is a guardian, but there is one person who really holds that space. When someone says something that is loaded with a lot of emotion, the guardian will often ring a bell for a brief period of silence to honour what was said. One ring of the bell or sound device calls for silence for about 15 seconds, and they ring it again to restart the sharing. Anyone in the circle can ask for the sound device to ask for silence. The person who asks for the bell to be rung often says why they requested it. This slows down the pace of the sharing, which is a good thing.

> Also, the guardian can ring the bell at the quarter turns of the circle to honour all the words spoken so far. This gives the circle time to process and integrate all that's been spoken. In Gather the Women circles, we always dedicate the energy of the circle at the end to some particular cause or persons. We often say in GTW, 'Ours is not the only way or a better way, ours is simply another way.'

Going back to the intention for your circle gathering will guide you in deciding whether others can support you in the circle dynamics and making the event feel special.

Finding a balance in circles

When people finally have a chance to be listened to and witnessed, big emotions do surface. However, talking circles can also be a place to connect with playfulness and joy. In circles there are often tears and raucous laughter in equal amounts even when the topic is sensitive, serious, challenging or taboo.

> People do need to go to those deep places, but also be reminded about how joyful life can be. It's not just permissible to have fun, but also celebrated and normalised. Lightness, joy and humour allows us to go way deeper, to open up more.
>
> *Benedict Beaumont*

It could be important to establish what brings people joy or fun or feelings of safety before going into challenging topics. Supporting people to recognise their existing resources is important. Perhaps sharing the practice of shaking could be introduced with some fun music like Taylor Swift's 'Shake It Off' song. Start with shaking the hands and arms, then add shaking a leg, switch to the other leg, even involve the whole body in the shaking. This can change the atmosphere in the room quickly. These sorts of activities act as pressure valves. Including movement breaks during the circle also supports people's nervous systems.

An activity that promotes connection is doing tree pose in a circle. At first, participants can balance alone, bringing one foot to the side of the other leg and bringing the palms together in front of the chest. They can take the arms up and out as branches and then reach out to the hands of the people on each side. Then they can play with supporting each other or sending a little wave around the circle of arms and trying to keep their balance.

● EXERCISE: DEEPENING YOUR LISTENING SKILLS

This exercise is another approach you can use to enhance your listening skills. It is embodied listening, based on the Focusing approach that was created by Gene Gendlin (see Gendlin 1997). It can be used in pairs to support people to reflect on their ability to listen when they feed back what they have heard.

Aim for three minutes each the first time you try this.

Person 1 – The Speaker: Take a moment to settle, with eyes closed if comfortable to do that, and then tune in to the body. You are creating a space to listen to what the body wants to communicate. Imagine sitting with a good friend: neither of you has to speak, but there is space and receptiveness if something comes up.

While you are receptive to the body, notice if a physical sensation arises in the body. Describe it aloud to the Listener in as much detail as possible. For example, 'I can feel a slight tension in my left shoulder. It feels like it's pulling my shoulder up. As I stayed with the sensation, it intensified, then started to release.'

Person 2 – The Listener: See if you can settle into a state of alert relaxation. Listen closely to what the speaker is saying. When there is a pause in their description, feed back the words that they used. For example, 'You felt tension in your left shoulder. It intensified, then started to release.'

If it's a few sentences, you might not be able to repeat back all that they said, so aim to feed back the essence of their description using their words. It's important not to change the description even if you think there is a more precise way to say it or put it into your words.

If you only remember the last few words, repeat those. In this example, 'Then started to release.' Having the exact words repeated makes the Speaker feel heard and witnessed.

Repeat the process until you've used the allotted time for the Listener.

The Speaker can ask two or three **clearing questions** to bring the person out of the embodied listening space (e.g. 'What did you eat for breakfast?'; 'What's your favourite colour?' Simple questions that are easily answered).

Swap over so that the Listener can be the Speaker and repeat the exercise.

When you explain this in a circle setting, you can invite the Speaker to clarify to their partner if they don't feed back quite right. For example, if the Listener said, 'It's yanking your shoulder up,' the Speaker might clarify with 'It's more that it's pulling my shoulder up.' This is good feedback for the Listener that they used their own word instead of the person's. It's also good practice for the Speaker to know the truth of their experience and be able to clarify it.

Then to bring people back into the circle, ask participants to share their experience of the process. They could share their own content of what they noticed, but not that of their partner.

This is a simplified version of the Focusing approach. For more information, go to www.focusing.org.uk.

Including quiet and marginalised voices

It is common for there to be people who are more quiet within a talking circle. They might feel more comfortable in one-to-one situations or prefer a listening role. See the exercise 'How to use listening partnerships' in this chapter for how to provide opportunities for speaking in pairs within the session. Listening partnerships enable an introduction to sharing that can then be brought back into the main circle.

During the main part of the circle, if you notice there are people who are not contributing, when there's a pause, say something like 'Would anybody who's not shared like to speak?' I might also use the people's names – for example, 'Anna, Esme, Priya. Would you like to say something about this? It's also fine if you're happy listening.'

For people who are not used to having a space to speak, it can be challenging to find the opportunity to come in, even with the guidelines of not talking over each other, aiming to be non-judgemental and so on. Their nervous system might be on high alert because of experiences where they tried to talk in the past and were knocked back or openly shut down.

In certain circles, you may wish specifically to uplift voices that are not usually heard. Julia attended a workshop about LGBTQIA+ inclusion in yoga and all the people from within the LGBTQIA+ community were invited to speak more than others. In this way, the learning within the circle was balanced well. The guidelines of the circle were clear that the intention was to elevate the voices of people within the LGBTQIA+ community. The event was also priced in a way that people from the LGBTQIA+ community paid less to attend and a donation was made to a charity that helped create more spaces for yoga specifically for that demographic.

A boy was there. He was about 19 years old. People were trying to explain the format to him. He asked, 'What do I say?' You could see him thinking, what do you mean, I share? You could see a lightbulb go off. It was wonderful to see. The circle is useful to break the usual social norms. You can share anything. You feel freer to really express yourself because you know it won't be commented upon.

Mark Walsh

If you realise that there are people missing from your circle, return to Chapter 3 on intention setting and read the section 'Inclusivity in circles'. For example, if you are running a women's circle and everyone looks the same in terms of age, ethnicity and financial health, perhaps you would like to think how you can invite a broader demographic to join. What would make them feel comfortable and able to attend and share in your circle? Diversity can lead to a richer experience for everyone.

When everyone is quiet

Sometimes you will ask people to share and there will be silence. Don't panic. Often time is needed to think about what to share, or perhaps someone doesn't want to jump in and stop someone else from talking. Take a few deep breaths and give yourself a moment to reflect too.

Usually, when you leave enough time, someone will start to speak. If still no-one speaks, you could offer your own experience as a way for people to have something to connect to. When you have already done an initial check-in so that everyone has said something aloud and shared the guidelines so the expectations for the way to communicate has been explained, it's unlikely that every person would be feeling too nervous to speak.

If it's a sensitive topic, more build-up may be required for attendees to feel comfortable. For example, Sophie Cleere, who runs sexuality circles, says, 'We do some settling work before and then it is gently guiding, so each structure [exercise] that we offer people goes a little bit deeper.'

Sharing your experience as the facilitator

Counsellors and psychotherapists generally do not share about their lives and experiences within a therapeutic encounter, so should a circle facilitator open up about themselves? From our experience, it depends. It depends on where the circle is happening, whether it's a one-off or a continued space and whether you have experience of the topic being talked about.

The depth of experience shared by people in a talking circle is usually directly related to how well the container has been created. If you are at a big festival, you might be able to have a fantastic container created by firm boundaries (e.g. people not coming in after the start of the circle, verbal agreement to the guidelines) that enables a deep sharing. Or you might decide you want to keep it lighter, where people can come and go, children can come in and out to look for their parents, and you put guidelines on a poster behind you. Your depth of sharing as a facilitator will most likely reflect the container too.

We feel strongly that there is a reciprocity in sharing your experience as a facilitator. If you are willing to share, it will build trust within the circle. If you are willing to be vulnerable, it will make it easier for others to be too. However, there is a line between sharing an experience that you've processed and one that is emotionally raw, which may tip you out of facilitation and into needing support yourself. If you are co-facilitating an established circle, there may be space for this, but reflect on how someone new might feel if they see the person who they thought was holding the space unravelling in front of them. As the facilitator, you are responsible for the container.

In situations where there is something that is new and full of raw emotion for you, it would be important to reach out for support elsewhere: talking therapies, supervision, a regular listening partnership or perhaps a different circle where you are a participant and not the facilitator.

> I find it edgy and difficult to judge what sharing I do. I am not in perimenopause; I am in a different space. I share how I am feeling, I share what is going on with me within the circle. I don't share my lived experience. I am sharing with a demographic I am no longer part of, so it would not be authentic for me to talk about my experience.
>
> *Kate Codrington (talking about menopause circles*
> *from the perspective of post-menopause)*

As Kate illustrates, it might be that you are facilitating a circle about something you have experienced in the past but is no longer your lived experience. This might be the case for people holding circles for new parents, who are parents themselves and can empathise, but are not in that intense stage of newborn life or experiencing the same context (e.g. parenting in the pandemic).

It might be that you're asked to facilitate a circle when you know nothing about the topic. This is certainly possible and may help the participants to consider new perspectives because of the questions you ask from a 'beginner's mind'. It may be clearer to see the dynamics within a talking circle if you are not an 'insider', and help bring awareness to the process rather than the content.

Your capacity to hold big emotions within the circle is equal to your capacity to hold your own emotions. For all of us, this is a work in progress.

CIRCLE STORY: FACILITATING BIG EMOTIONS

Content warning: In this story there is talk of attempting suicide. Please speak to the Samaritans for support if needed: www.samaritans. org.

Tessa shares an experience from her women's circle:

> I'll share with you one of the stand-out moments in facilitating talking circles. It was a challenging situation to hold and very difficult for the person concerned at the time. It was also a turnaround moment in the person's life for the better.
>
> The women's circle had been running for years and this lady had been a regular attendee for some months. She was at a time of real transition in her life, which she had shared openly in the circle before. On this particular night, the circle started and we were doing an initial round when she shared that she had tried to kill herself the night before.
>
> I paused and let it sink in. I then responded, saying her name and that I was glad she had come and could share that. Something shifted in that moment. I think it was because it was a very different response from the one she'd received from people that morning.
>
> I didn't ask her what had led her to that action but asked her how she was now and if there was anything she needed from us. She said that she just wanted to be in this circle and have company. Of course, her disclosure affected all of us, and people spoke about their gladness that she was there, her courage in sharing what happened and that she wasn't alone in experiencing mental health issues.
>
> At the end, I checked in with her about people she could call on and what resources she had in place going forward. Years later after she moved away, we're still in touch and she says the circle was pivotal to her moving forward: 'I will never ever forget the kindness I experienced when I felt I couldn't talk to anyone else.'

This may seem like a daunting scenario to contemplate as a circle facilitator, but think about how you would act in any other situation: hopefully, as a compassionate person doing their best. Setting the guidelines at the beginning of the circle that people are responsible for themselves is important. She had judged that she was ready to attend the circle and share what had happened.

We invite you as a facilitator to have somewhere you are supported – particularly if situations like this happen, but also as best practice to enable resilience, a sustainable circle and your growth as a circle holder.

If you already have experience of holding space in other contexts (e.g. managing meetings, conducting interviews or appraisals, teaching, counselling), you might find that you have skills that transfer to managing circle dynamics. The next exercise will support your reflection on circle skills whether you are new to facilitation or experienced.

EXERCISE: BUILDING YOUR CIRCLE SKILLS

Take some time to consider these questions. Writing down or drawing responses will support your reflection.

- Where can you practise (new) phrases that help you manage the circle dynamics? (Both for helping quieter participants and for guiding dominant ones.)

- How does it feel to use timing to provide a container for people speaking? (If it feels uncomfortable, can you reframe so that you recognise you're meeting the needs of everyone present?)

- How comfortable are you with silence? How comfortable are you with someone crying and not rushing in with tissues? (Exposure is most helpful here – it gets easier the more you're in the situation.)

- How much are you willing to share your experience in the circle? What feels appropriate for this setting?

- Who can you ask to be a regular listening partner?

- Is there an online or in-person circle you can attend as a participant?

- Would formal supervision be helpful?

Return to these questions periodically as the answers may change. Your skills will grow as you have more practice being a facilitator.

There is an art to circle holding: of creating a structure that provides a strong container and at the same time being fluid enough to let the talking go where it is most helpful. This comes from practice. Reflecting on circle dynamics and how you handle them with other circle holders or with a mentor will accelerate your facilitation capacity.

In the next chapter, we consider how to close the circle and support people returning to their everyday life.

CHAPTER 11

Closing the Circle

You notice that you're coming towards the end of the time and yet the flow of talk is the strongest it's been. Respecting that some will need to be off promptly, you ask that we check in with everyone as we prepare to close. Going around the circle, everyone has a chance to speak about the experience of being in the circle today. There is a feeling of something having transformed through the time spent together. People start to move and collect their belongings; some gravitate towards each other and talk.

If you like, close your eyes after reading this sentence, take a slow breath in and out, connect with now.

Closing the circle is as important as the opening. It is part of the container that supports people to feel held through the circle process to its completion. It is a signal that this special space is coming to an end. We recommend having a clear start and finish time. It is important to respect the finishing time because people may have planned other activities afterwards or need to get home to bed to be prepared for the next day.

In a two-hour circle, we recommend allowing about 15 minutes for closing the talking circle. Sharing what time it is and drawing attention to how much time has passed helps people prepare for the end of the session. Having one more round of sharing in the circle can be a wonderful way to integrate what has happened and support reflection on the process. For example, you might ask:

- What will you take away from the circle today?

- How are you feeling as we come to the end of the circle?

- What small kindness can you take into your life?

- What can you do tomorrow to remind yourself of what we've talked about?

Depending on how many people are in circle and how much time you have left, you might want to set a time limit of one or two minutes, with a chime to let people know when that time has passed. If you're really short of time, asking people to share one or two words to sum up how they're feeling can work well.

Kate Codrington shared:

> Closing is about integrating back into everyday life. It has to be grounded in something real. You want to give value to people so they are able to take the value into their everyday life. It's also a bridge: 'Here I am in this lovely, fluffy circle, but what am I going to do tomorrow?' How you take that feeling into everyday life.

Ideas for closing

If journalling has been part of the circle, you might first ask the participants to go back to the journal to reflect on what they have learnt about themselves during the circle, or what insights they will take away with them. They could then verbally share one aspect if they want to in the final round of sharing. Journalling is a wonderful way of beginning to process what has come up and enable reflection after the event has finished.

Perhaps you have access to a fire and can invite people to write out anything that they wish to let go of. Perhaps they saw during the circle things in their life that are no longer serving them. They can fold over the piece of paper if they wish to keep it to themselves, or speak it aloud to the group. Burning the words can create a symbolic opening for change. For an extra-special circle, sourcing 'flash paper' or 'fire paper' that burns in a flash and seems to disappear before your eyes is worth the extra cost.

When you have lit a candle at the start of the circle, in the closing round it feels poignant to blow out the candle after you have spoken your final sharing. If this is what you're planning, make sure that your tealights will last the length of the circle! Tessa loves to put the candles on a circular mirror so that the light is reflected out into the space, with a bigger, central candle to light the individual ones from.

Closing with listening partnerships

You may want to have people listening to each other in pairs, as described in Chapter 10. Using partner work in the closing segment would be useful if there is someone who has been reluctant to speak during the main part of the circle time.

Prompts could be:

- My takeaway from today is...

- At the end of the circle, I feel...

- Through listening to others, I have learnt...

We would still encourage a one-word check-in with the whole circle to provide a sense of togetherness as you finish.

Using touch for connection

You may want to bring touch into the circle where it is appropriate. A simple way of doing this if you are sitting close enough is to have everyone's left palm facing upwards and the right palm facing downwards. Then around the circle everyone's palms are connected. Taking three breaths in this position can be enough to anchor that feeling of belonging.

A fun way of connecting through the hands that can also be used with children is to bring the fingertips together, or palms, as people wish, with hands turned out to the people either side. Then the facilitator can add a little push through one hand to create a wave around the circle. This often leads to giggling amongst kids as the wave disappears and random waves appear!

If it's a small enough circle that you can reach together into the circle, you can all place a hand into the centre, higgledy-piggledy one over the other. With children you might wiggle the fingers and make imaginary stardust fly through the air as you take your arm back.

If you've been holding a circle with movement, making a human mandala is lovely. With up to eight people, you can move in closer (if there's no centrepiece) and put your right feet together, with the leg straight. The left knee is bent and relaxed to the side. Then you can reach out to bring each others' palms together or have fun trying to reaching into the middle with first the right hand and then the left hand (see Figure 7.2).

If people brought objects to create a centrepiece, remind them to retrieve their precious belongings before they leave. However, if the centrepiece is created out of natural objects, you could symbolically close the circle by gathering the materials that are laid out on and throwing them on to the fire or into a stream (if this is appropriate environmentally). This echoes the sand mandalas created in Tibetan cultures that can take months to intricately lay out and then get brushed away in a moment on completion. Everything is impermanent!

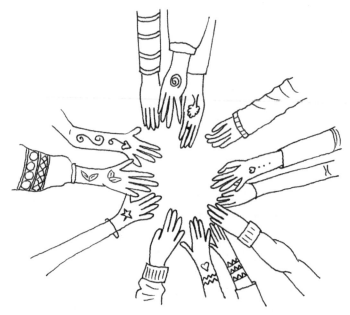

Figure 11.1 Hands with henna designs at circle's close

Sharing words and sounds together

You may have set words that you repeat every time that have a meaning for your particular community, or that you've made up and have become tradition. For example, you might say, 'We've closed our circle and we remain connected until next time. May you listen carefully and be listened to with the same care.'

In yoga circles, people might repeat together, 'Om shanti, shanti, shanti', calling for peace. If using words in another language, it's important to explain what they mean and the context in which they are used. We sometimes use the repetition of 'Om' in our yoga classes because it is so beautiful to hear the sound of many voices overlapping, but always offer that people can hum instead if they don't connect with 'Om'.

Henika Patel shared:

In circle, usually we are working with a particular theme which is either intentional or emerges naturally. The last part of the circle we share a song or mantra. I either play a recording, sing myself or invite the circle to join. It is a beautiful integration to sing or dance together to close circle: to share the space that the mantra or music holds and to thank the ancestors for the practices we've experienced.

You could also use a sound such as hand chimes being struck three times to mark the beginning and end of the circle. Some of Tessa's favourite memories of the women's circle are sitting round a fire singing songs together at the end, including the one below. Singing together often feels more comfortable once connection has been made and deepened.

Deep down, deep down, deep down in our hearts
Deep down, deep down, deep down in our hearts
Tessa we love you, deep down in our hearts.
Deep down, deep down, deep down in our hearts
Deep down, deep down, deep down in our hearts
[Next person's name] we love you, deep down in our hearts.

Artist unknown

Another one Julia loves is:

May all mothers know that they are loved
And may all sisters know that they are strong
And may all daughters know that they are worthy/beautiful/powerful
That the circle of women may live on
That the fire of the goddess may burn on
Waheya waheya waheya

*Nalini Blossom, Circle of Women (permission granted
to share lyrics, see www.naliniblossom.com)*

Julia shared:

I loved this song so much that after sitting in circle at the Sun and Moon Festival with my young daughter we sang it together for weeks afterwards at bedtime! She even wrote the lyrics down on my birthday card that year.

If you have the confidence and skills to include singing or live music, they can be profound experiences for people and create lasting memories.

As you can see, there are different ways of marking the ending, but it's important to be clear that the talking circle has formally finished. Often people want to chat in an informal way afterwards but don't want to break the guidelines that have been laid out.

Example: Red Thread ceremony

For special occasions, like waiting for a baby to be born or a person moving away, holding a Red Thread ceremony at the close of the circle can feel very special. Of course, you can choose any colour thread you like that is relevant to the occasion. The idea probably came from the Hindu festival of Rakshabandhan where sisters tie a protective thread around the right wrist of their brothers. The word 'rakshabandhan' means 'tie of protection'.

Sitting in a circle, pass the ball of cotton thread to each person, winding it around each person's right wrist (or ankle if it will be a problem at work). Once the thread has gone all the way around the circle, say some words about the occasion. For example, for a mother blessing, you might say:

Until your baby arrives, we will be thinking of you every time we see the thread around our wrists. We will be sending all our best wishes for the birthing journey and giving our support after the baby arrives. Only when we hear news that the baby has arrived will we cut off the thread, to mark the baby's separation from you with the cutting of the umbilical cord. Know that you are held in community.

For someone moving away from the circle, you could offer the words:

With this thread around your wrist, remember that we have been connected through sharing in the circle over the years and are physically connected by the thread now. Our connection is still there as you move away to a new beginning. Every time you see the thread, know that we are thinking of you too.

You can also ask others to contribute words too. Once all the words have been shared, pass a pair of scissors around the circle to cut the thread between people's wrists. Gather up the ends and circle them around the wrist with just enough to tie off. Invite people's neighbours to do the tying as it's very tricky to do yourself.

It's important that the thread is thick cotton rather than wool.

Wool will start to sag as it gets wet and will fall off. Buying thick cotton from a craft or haberdashery shop will ensure that it lasts as long as possible.

You can also invite people to ceremonially cut off the thread when they hear news of the baby arriving, for example. Perhaps they can tie it on a tree in their garden or local park, keep it in a box of mementos or secure it in a diary. Others will wait until the thread eventually falls off by itself.

The Red Thread ceremony is a symbolic way of marking the connection between people in the circle and, where appropriate, wishing them protection for their next journey. Julia shares a memory of this ceremony:

> I remember us all singing a song we had learned as the thread was passed from person to person, and for many weeks afterwards until the bracelet eventually became worn and came off, I would think of the special time I had with the group and it would make me smile.

If you are running a series of circles with a clear beginning and end date for a defined group, the Red Thread ceremony can be a great way to create a special atmosphere at the end of the final session. It has also been done successfully with groups at the end of a weekend or week retreat or training together.

Remember, there's no one way of closing a circle. Benedict Beaumont shared:

> I might play something fun to finish off with. Dancing round to some music to end the circle – a dance can be a really nice way to end a circle – uplifting movement and people will naturally drift off and conversations will happen.

As long as it's clear to the participants what is happening and when the circle has ended, so that they can choose whether to stay or socialise, you can finish with something uplifting like dance.

Including informal time

It's advisable to factor in chat time as people gather their belongings, and it creates a transition back to the outer world. You can explicitly say how much time there is for this element so that you don't become resentful of people overstaying their welcome in the venue!

When Tessa ran her women's circle in a yurt in a field, she would pack up as people were chatting and then say that it was time to go. When the circle was in her living room at home, people were asked to chat in the room and then quietly exit through her hallway so as not to wake up her children upstairs. Be clear in guiding people in what you need them to do according to your constraints with time and the environment.

It might be that you include refreshments within the circle and have them available at the end too to support socialising and mingling. Food is a grounding mechanism as well as a chance to encourage social interaction. In mother and daughter circles, Tessa always includes time for the girls to have squash and snacks, and time to play together, while the mums have tea and a chance to talk to each other. This helps bonds to be created and for offshoots like playdates and picnics to be organised. Julia will often include the timing for this in her introduction:

> The circle ends at HH:MM. Please feel free to stay for 15 minutes afterwards while I pack up the space.

or:

> The circle ends at HH:MM. The Zoom will stay open for 15 minutes afterwards if you would like to ask any questions or talk about anything that has come up during the group.

Remember to tell people when the next circle is, and if you don't already have their contact details, collect these so that you can remind them. If you are new to holding circles or want to check in with people's experience, you can collect feedback as part of the closing circle or afterwards. For example, the closing round might be 'What did you most enjoy and what did you find most challenging about being in the circle?' Or you could ask people to write their thoughts on post-it notes before they leave so that they can express their feelings anonymously.

Particularly if it is a short gathering, the closing can simply involve taking note of the time, saying when the next meeting will be and how to join.

When the circle has finished and everyone has left, your process of closing is still under way. We will talk about this more in the next chapter.

● EXERCISE: CONSCIOUSLY CLOSING

How you close the circle is as important as how you open it. Read through these two scenarios and imagine how they would make you feel as a participant rather than the facilitator. Write down your thoughts.

First scenario: You're sitting in a lively circle and the talk is in full flow. You glance at the clock and are surprised to see that two and a half hours have gone by. You were expecting the gathering to last two hours from something you saw on the website, but the facilitator hasn't mentioned what time it will finish.

The talking continues for another half an hour before someone asks what time the event will end. The circle holder says, 'Since this has overrun, let's finish now so people who need to leave can. Thank you so much for coming, everyone.' Talking breaks into pairs and many people still sit for another three-quarters of an hour.

Second scenario: You're sitting in a lively circle and the talk is in full flow. The facilitator says that there are ten minutes left before the official close of the circle and that they'd like to slowly start winding things up. A pause is introduced, with a couple of minutes to reflect about the experience of being in circle today. Then everyone is invited to speak for one minute, with a chime marking when their turn ends. Some speak for the full minute, others don't.

Then there is an invitation to look around the circle at each other and someone is asked to blow out the candle in the centrepiece. Everyone knows from the joining instructions in the email beforehand that there's up to 30 minutes for socialising, but you don't have to stay for this part. The facilitator sees each person to the door as a final personal check-in.

After reflecting on how it would feel as a participant to attend these circles, turn your attention to how you would manage the first scenario if you'd lost track of time, and how it would feel to stop the flow of talk in the second scenario. What do you imagine the closing component of your circle will look like?

How you respond to these scenarios might depend on your personality, your circumstances (e.g. if you need to leave on time for another appointment or for childcare reasons) and previous experience of navigating social situations and even trauma. Next we have a story from someone who specialises in closing the circle.

CIRCLE STORY: CELEBRATION DAY FOR GIRLS

The Celebration Day for Girls (CDG) were created by Jane Bennett. Tessa runs one each year for girls aged 10–12 years old. It provides an opportunity for girls to learn more about their menstrual cycle and period products, and normalises talking about bodies.

At the end of the day is a wonderful ceremony where the mums (or female caregivers) recognise that their daughters are embarking on a new stage in their lives. (They might or might not have already started their period.) It provides a special way of closing the day that makes the event really memorable.

The girls decorate themselves with henna or biodegradable glitter. Tessa then takes them out into the corridor and asks them to stand tall and be really proud about openly learning about their bodies. Tessa invites them to walk out with confidence as they approach this new stage of their lives. The mums receive their daughters and present them with something that they made earlier in the day.

The mothers have already been prepped with how to receive their daughters and so Tessa beats her hand drum, bringing a sense of occasion. The daughters walk out to meet their mothers and be presented with the special item and with special words. Usually some happy tears are shed by the mums!

Then the singing begins, going around the circle addressing each person with the words 'deep down, deep down in our hearts' (see earlier in this chapter for the full words). When you are named, your heart swells with warmth. It happens to me every time.

Not everyone has access to ceremony and ritual nowadays. Introducing them can make gatherings feel special, enhance belonging through shared experience and add to the container of the circle.

After the event

For most circle holders, there will be some packing away and tidying up time after people have left. If you have a dedicated space for your circle where you can leave it set up, lucky you! We recommend taking some time to close your own process. In Chapter 5, we suggested ways to prepare your nervous system so that you would be ready to welcome circle attendees in a grounded way. It might be that your nervous system needs grounding at the end of the gathering too!

Tessa finds that it takes her an hour after holding a two-hour circle to be ready for bed (the women's circle runs 7.30–9.30 p.m.). From being very attentive to listening to people's experiences and guiding the dynamics, then reflecting on what happened, a process of settling happens.

You might also find a few days after the event that you want to journal about the experience of holding the circle. Avoid writing down the content of what people talked about to maintain confidentiality. Reflecting on how you could have managed a situation better or where you felt uncomfortable may provide learning.

Mentoring or supervision is another option that can provide you support to develop your facilitation skills or to reflect on the process, particularly if you are holding space with challenging experiences. Remember that a listening partnership (see Chapter 10) with another circle holder can provide a cost-effective option too.

The end of the journey: When and how to end your circle group

You may decide that your circle will run for a specific length of time. It could be a circle created for a specific purpose that will run for a number of consecutive weeks, or a year-long journey. If there is a specific end date, inform the participants of that date at the start of the process; you may decide to create something special for the final circle.

A circle could also be set up as a regular event with no end date planned. When you have been running a circle for a long time, it might be hard to imagine stopping it, because the gathering has become a fixture in the community. If you feel that it is time for you to move on, you could ask for a co-collaborator to come on board for handover sessions. If there is no-one willing, it might be that you need to stop it completely, and having a final circle would close the container for good.

The Red Thread practice above could be a way you might choose to end a circle you have been running for a specific time. Allowing for a special circle that marks the end can give a feeling of completion and can also give the people who have been part of the circle the opportunity to express their gratitude and needs for their next step.

If you are running a circle for a specific demographic, you might make a special time for those who are moving out of that space. This could be because they have grown out of an age group or they are no longer part of the demographic (e.g. no longer perimenopausal or a new parent). Honouring the transition out of a talking circle is important and could be something people enjoy, and ceremony can create a beautiful memory to savour.

In the next few chapters, we look in more detail at embodiments in circles, complementary activities and working with children.

CHAPTER 12

Embodiment in Circles: Movement, Meditation and Mindfulness

Imagine you've spent all day in your head, busy thinking and taking in information from different media. At last, here is a chance to be in a space where phones are switched off and you can listen to one person at a time. There is time to connect with how your body is feeling by slowing down and soothing the nervous system. You show up in the world in a different way.

In previous chapters, we've mentioned practices that connect with the body and settle the nervous system. This may seem strange in a guide about talking and listening circles, but it is a part of the process in enabling people to feel comfortable enough to speak freely. The authors of this book are yoga teachers, teaching continually to facilitate people's connection to their own bodies, and have weaved circle time into our yoga classes.

The value of bringing physical awareness into circle time is that we are able to settle more easily and listen with more focus once we have given our nervous system the opportunity to settle. If we are tackling a challenging topic in a listening circle, giving the body the opportunity to release pent-up energy can be really valuable. This is particularly the case when working with children who are required to sit still at school.

The embodiment tools we share later in the chapter are easy to practise and incorporate into your circle even if you are not trained in movement.

A note to yoga teachers and movement professionals
You may have joined us because you already have a tool box full of meditation, movement and relaxation skills. If that is the case, a circle is a great place to share your practices. You might start by seeing whether it is possible to change the structure of your teaching space so that you are in a circle with your students rather than at the front of the room with your students following you. Notice what this does to the feeling of the space and how you see each other. Your students will no longer be one in front of the other but will be able to make eye contact with each other.

You may then choose to use some of the opening practices we shared in Chapter 7 to open your yoga/movement circle. You then might close your class with some of the practices described in Chapter 11. We find that changing our classes to this way of practising is more intimate and brings students into community with each other. Rather than entering class, practising and leaving without even learning each other's names, opportunity has arisen for a new way of being together and for friendships to flourish.

The body is an incredible part of the self, which can provide much insight. Rather than being a vehicle to carry yourself around in, it is very much part of the process of heightening self-awareness. You might have heard people in a circle gathering say things like 'As you were speaking, I felt a tension in my chest,' 'Thinking about that topic, I feel like a lead weight' or 'Thank you for this circle, I feel so much lighter in my body now.' This connection of feelings to the body is really important.

A psychotherapist called Gene Gendlin wondered why some of his therapy clients became better and some didn't. He spent time analysing the transcripts from therapy sessions and found that those who used interoception, their felt sense (as in the examples above), were the ones who became better. Interoception is the awareness of our body, whether it's butterflies before an interview or the feeling of your heart physically being broken after a relationship break-up.

Tessa finds that in the embodied listening that she facilitates for people who've experienced birth trauma, they may have been having counselling for months or even years, and yet something new will emerge when space is created to simply be with the body. One form of embodied listening formalised by Gene Gendlin is Focusing, and this can be learnt by anyone (see Gendlin 1997).

Another reason that this is helpful in a talking circle setting is that using a practice that settles people's nervous systems will usually support a deeper level of connection between people. Using ways to help someone connect with the experience of being in their body can shift the talking from a superficial level to a deeper level of insight and may introduce a different way of feeling in your body while in relationship with others. Conversely, it can also help someone to know if what is being talked about makes them feel uncomfortable.

When we connect to our bodies, we can feel how words land in a way that we didn't expect. If we play with tightening and releasing those parts of the body that are commonly affected by stress (our mouths, tummies and shoulders are good examples), we are more likely to notice if they react during a talking circle. If you have ever been in a room where someone has been shouting, it is possible to feel the negative energy created and notice how that made us feel. The same is true when we introduce a practice that is calming to the nervous system. Something as simple as placing your hand on your heart can bring a sense of calm and connect us to a gentler way of communicating.

Examples of embodiment practices

We offer here some of our favourites out of the thousands of embodiment practices that you could use. If you are not a movement teacher or somatic practitioner or someone else who teaches embodied practices, we recommend you try the ones below and see which you're most comfortable with. Practise something thoroughly so that you're sharing from a place of experience. Also refer back to the embodiment practice and the resting practice in Chapter 7, described in the exercise 'Examples of settling practices'.

● EXERCISE: BUTTERFLY HOLD

Sit with your left hand on the right side of your chest and your right hand on the left side of your chest, like the wings of a butterfly. You can hook the thumbs around each other in the centre. Tap the fingers of the left hand gently on the chest and then tap the fingers of the right hand gently on the other side of the chest.

Choose a rhythm that is soothing to you, not too fast and not too slow, not too gentle and not too hard. That might be enough to focus on. You could also pay attention to your breathing once the tapping is under way. Breathe in and breathe out for the same length in a way that is a little deeper than usual for you, but comfortable and sustainable.

The idea with this alternating bilateral stimulation is that your brain is focused on the repetitive sensations and stays in the present, while realising that this stimulus is not threatening. This deactivates the flight and fight reaction of our sympathetic nervous system.

You can also try reaching a little further across to the upper arms, left hand to the top of the right arm and right hand to the top of the left arm. You can either gently squeeze, alternating from side to side, or stroke slowly downwards, alternating left and right. This is called havening: you are creating your own nervous system haven!

Notice how it feels to receive your own touch and how the body responds. You can stop at any time.

This could be used as a settling practice before moving into the main topic, and repeated if the talking becomes very charged or to support integration at the end of the circle. One of Tessa's circle holder trainees works in a prison and said that the male inmates would not want to use their hands on their chest or arms. Tessa suggested tapping on the thighs instead (left hand on left leg, right hand on right leg) and tapping alternately to create the soothing rhythm.

If you have the expertise, you could share a yoga nidra (yoga sleep) practice. Yoga nidra is a wonderful restorative practice that can be used for relaxation or meditation. It is an embodiment practice because guidance about breathing and noticing physical sensation is commonly included, but also because a rotation around the body is standard. We recommend finding out more about practices such as yoga nidra you could use to start a circle.

The next extended exercise is to show how you can start a talking and listening circle from an embodied practice. The womb might not be relevant to your specific demographic, but we hope that you can use it as an example of how you can create an enquiry about any part of the body.

● EXERCISE: CONNECTING TO THE FUNCTIONAL AND EMOTIONAL BODY

These practices can be used with a variety of body parts as a springboard for circle discussion.

Heart/womb/gut connection

This practice is for connecting to the womb or womb space. It can be healing for those who have had their womb removed and for those who have experienced challenges connected to their womb. In mixed spaces, Julia shares this practice with the option to connect to the gut as an alternative to the womb.

1. Share a settling practice to ensure everyone in the circle is sitting comfortably either on the floor, using blocks, meditation cushions or stools, or a chair. If sitting on a chair, ensure that their feet are firmly in contact with the ground, or with blocks if their legs are too short to touch the ground.

2. Invite those in the circle to either close their eyes or allow a soft gaze downwards. Either alternative is fine and it is likely they will close their eyes at some point in the practice even if they have chosen to keep them open.

3. Invite them to bring their left hand to their heart and to cover the left with their right. If you model this for them, then participants who are unsure can copy you without feeling self-conscious about whether they are getting the practice 'right'.

4. Take time and space for them to notice the coming and going of their breath – they are likely to feel this underneath their hands. You can use words like 'Notice the feeling of your body beneath your hands. Can you notice the texture of your clothing under your hands? Is it possible to feel the movement in your body as it breathes?'

5. Invite the participants to bring their attention to their heart. You can then invite them to bring to mind something nice, a pleasant memory or feeling, and to notice whether they can sense how that feels in their heart. If that feels okay, they can choose to bring to mind something or someone that they love.

6. It can be helpful here to provide examples – maybe a food they love to eat or a person who is special to them. Providing options allows them to choose whether to keep their feelings light or to go a little deeper.

7. You can then invite them to notice any feeling in their heart. Once they have done this, it is likely that they will begin to notice the physical feelings associated with the heart. Note that whatever those participating feel is totally valid and that includes them not feeling anything physically. All experience is valid experience and there is no right or wrong.

You could choose to end the practice here and bring everyone back into circle. You could use the words:

I invite you to gently bring your attention back to your breathing. Have an awareness of the movement that occurs in your body as you breathe. Gently lower your hands to your lap, and if your eyes have been closed you can open them with the gaze downward. Slowly and in your own time, begin to look around the room; look up at the ceiling/sky, down to the ground beneath you, and press your hands into your chair/the floor. Then come back into circle.

At this point you may wish to look around the circle and make eye contact with those who choose to. This helps relocate them in space. At this point, you could invite people to share their experience of the practice.

If you choose to continue to the full practice, you could use words similar to these:

Now as you breathe in, keep the right hand over the left at the heart and as you breathe out, lower the right hand to the womb space or gut. With each in-breath return the right hand to the heart and with each out-breath allow the right hand to move down to the womb space/gut.

Look round the circle to establish whether most of the participants are following the practice. It is okay if some are choosing not to: when we use invitational language, it is so that people can make their own choice and that might mean that they do not follow the embodiment practice.

You now have the option to either continue the practice in this way or keep the left hand over the heart and the right hand over the womb space/gut and move your attention from heart to womb/gut and back again.

Once you have established whichever practice works for you, you may wish to connect to your womb space.

Depending on the group you are with, there are various ways to connect to the womb. Julia has shared this practice with:

- pregnancy circles

- perimenopause and menopause circles

- wider groups including women of various ages

- mixed-gender group settings.

In pregnancy circles you may wish to use language that could enable those present to connect with their babies. For example:

> Send love from your heart to your baby, floating in the womb space. Feel the connection between your heart and your baby. You might even be able to feel your baby's movements as you sit here taking time and space to connect to your baby.

In postnatal circles it can be helpful to use language that brings connection to the womb as a place that has been home to their baby for so long. Maybe bringing thankfulness to that space. Often there can be a feeling of discomfort around the size and shape of the belly after childbirth, so reconnecting to the womb space postnatally in this way can be helpful.

In perimenopause and menopause circles you may have created time and space to talk about this time and there may be those in the circle who have experienced:

- miscarriage

- abortion

- womb removal

- childbirth

- not have experienced childbirth.

Using careful language, it is possible to connect to any of the above themes.

With regard to connection to the gut, the theme of 'gut feeling' and intuition can be explored.

Once you have explored any of the themes above through the practice of placing the hand on the heart and the womb (space) or gut, invite participants to bring their attention back to the hands and the connection between the hands and the heart and womb, and then to return both hands to the heart.

Julia has found over many years of sharing practices where a connection is made to the physical body that profound sharing can take place in circle time afterwards. Over the years, those in circle have shared their experiences of baby loss, passing childbearing age without having children, hysterectomy, breast operations due to the experience of cancer, connecting to creativity and projects, finding the next step when stuck, connecting with the challenges of painful periods, irritable bowels, postnatal bodies and many other experiences.

The use of physical touch together with words connecting to emotion and memory can be very powerful. Sometimes in circle time tears come as participants share or listen to others' testimony. While it is helpful to have a box of tissues to hand, allowing the tears and offering a smile and the words 'Thank you for sharing' is often all that is required. No fixing. No advice. Simply space holding.

Incorporating the body in our circle work can bring benefits outside of circle time. If we are given space to notice how our bodies feel in response to what someone else is saying in a circle, we may be more likely to notice those sensations in our daily lives. We have found that practising embodiment within a circle can sometimes help us be less reactive in our lives. We are more likely to notice strong emotions without immediately acting upon them.

Common questions about embodiment practices
What if people are embarrassed to move in front of others?
Sometimes facilitators are worried about people feeling embarrassed about joining in with movement. Communicate what practices will be included in your marketing so that people are not surprised. If people are okay with closing their eyes, this can take a lot of the intensity out of trying a new physical movement. If there is space and the venue can be set up comfortably with cushions and something to cover the floor, you can ask people to lie down to try practices. If you are inviting people to lie down, heads could be positioned in the centre of the circle, with feet to the outside, so that people feel less watched.

Start simple. Even drawing attention to the breath can have a huge impact on how someone feels, and there is nothing noticeably happening from the outside. Also consider that how you model the practice influences how it is received. If you are totally comfortable with doing it and present it as an experiment to see how the practice affects them, they may feel that they have nothing to lose. Less is more when it comes to introducing movement and embodiment practices, so use the concept of titration (tiny drops of experiencing such practice) and offer small practices with check-ins afterwards to see how they're being received. It's also okay for someone to opt out and watch.

Do I need training to include embodiment in circles?

You do not need training to include simple practices like noticing the breath or noticing your body. It is important that you are practising these things if you are going to share them, and you may wish to train when you see the benefits. Find resources like the exercises in this book or recorded meditations that you can use.

If you are trained in movement, such as yoga, tai chi or dance, you may wish to create a hybrid event. For example, in a two-hour session you could have one hour of movement and one hour of circle time. Particularly if you are introducing the concept of circle to your existing movement clients, offering the activity they associate with you with the circle process may be more attractive.

For this model, you will need sufficient space for the movement practice and may need to specify what type of clothing people would feel most comfortable in. You can bring in a circle of chairs after the movement or sit on the floor with enough props to feel comfortable. Think about how you can accommodate those that may not want to sit on the floor for extended periods.

Do I have to include embodiment in my circle?

You don't need to explicitly include it, but people's bodies and nervous systems will be reacting to being in a circle gathering. By guiding people to notice this and including simple practices around awareness, you are supporting their reflective process and their comfort to be in the space.

Could movement or breathwork be triggering for people?

It is important that you say in marketing whether movement or breathwork will be included in the circle. If people know that this might be triggering of past trauma for them, they can decide that it's not the circle for them or tell you that it might be an issue (without needing to tell you why).

Always offer an option to keep eyes open and provide choices. Certain positions can be triggering for people, but if you have said that they can choose an alternative position, you are giving them agency to do what is right for them. Breathwork can be challenging when someone has experienced trauma because it usually involves controlling the breath. Depending on whether a nervous system is in flight/fight or shutdown/freeze, different types of breathing would be indicated. Again, offering that people can always stay with an awareness of their normal breath without trying to change anything or noticing something neutral in their body (e.g. usually sensations in the feet are neutral) is helpful here.

The guideline of 'taking responsibility for yourself' is important here. Encourage people to choose the option that feels right for them. With any embodiment practice, it is essential to give options when instructing people how to do it so that they can opt out. If someone is not used to connecting with their body, or their body feels like an unsafe place, they need to feel that they have the option not to join in. Titration might mean that these practices become more available to them over time.

In yoga for trauma, simple movements are used to move from raw emotion to a state where the nervous system moves away from flight or fight. *Overcoming Trauma through Yoga: Reclaiming Your Body* by David Emerson and Elizabeth Hopper (2011) is a good starting point for learning about the profound effect of movement and how to provide choice when sharing movement practices.

There is a spectrum of enquiries into embodiment, from noticing the breath to working with sexual touch. Some circle holders are experts in holding space for explorations around sensuality and consent, and should have taken extra steps in creating a container for this type of work.

CIRCLE STORY: POSITIVE SEXUALITY

Sophie Cleere has been supporting people to explore their sexual being through workshops and retreats, having been on her own journey of embodiment:

> For a lot of my time as a yoga teacher, I wasn't connected to my body. I feel that most of the time when I was practising ashtanga seriously, there was a lot of disembodiment.
>
> The thing that changed everything for me was the conscious sexuality work. It wasn't about making a shape or my body needing to be in a certain way. It was much more about how does it feel in my body? What does it feel like in my body when I am relaxed? What does it

feel like in my body when I am shut down? What does it feel like in my body when I feel juicy or aroused?

It really began when I started holding space with my partner. That is when I got brave and we started holding space together. My exploration with sensuality and sexuality and embodiment taught me so much because it is such a confronting thing: it is something that is amazing, and can also be traumatising, and can cause pain, and can be used against people.

We are always beginning and ending in circle, so there is an opportunity for people to check in and say how they are feeling.

The most important thing from the beginning is creating that container of safety. In terms of what that looks like in a conscious sexuality retreat, for example, that would start when I speak to someone on the phone before they come. Because if someone isn't in the right place to do it, or they are not the right person for it, you have that space to find out. You are building that relationship and that trust early on.

We say, 'Come with someone – so you have someone who has got your back.' That [creation of a container] begins before people come to the event. Someone might be very new to the work. Coming with a partner or friend is really helpful. We know people who run events like ours who are much less strict, but it is very important to us that we manage our space meticulously.

In summary, including embodiment in circle time can be incredibly valuable and it can form the main focus of the gathering. To do this, you need to have experience of embodiment yourself, be clear in your marketing what will be covered and create as strong a container for the circle as you can. This may include talking individually with people before they attend to understand and manage their expectations.

In the next chapter, we look at other complementary activities that you may include in a talking and listening circle.

CHAPTER 13

Complementary Activities

Although the focus of the circle is respectful talking and deep listening, you decide to include a mindful activity in the event. You notice this supports those that are less talkative to feel engaged throughout the gathering. Those that are talkative have something to occupy them and there are more spaces for others to share.

Did you know that, traditionally, a midwife would knit while she waited for babies to be born and keep an eye on labour out of the corner of her eye? This meant that she was close at hand, but also that the mother didn't feel scrutinised or that something needed to happen imminently.

For the same reason, introducing a mindful activity can occupy people enough that the focus on someone talking is softened. It can either soothe the nervous system or, if you have a group where people are in a state of freeze or numbness, it can gently upregulate. Anything sensory is wonderful here – for example, colouring in, sorting seeds/pulses/lentils, using natural objects to make a mandala and using clay to make something. The number of mindful colouring books on the market in recent years is testament to the connection between keeping the hands and mind focused and a sense of calm and ease.

These complementary activities can also be used when the circle is about a more sensitive topic. Choosing an activity to keep eyes and hands busy will support people to share experiences despite the potential for feeling more vulnerable.

Ideas for using crafts and activities

If you are inviting everyone to take part in the craft or activity, it needs to be something that all will be able to learn how to do or contribute to, and achievable in the time available. It is well worth having a trial run with friends to see whether it is possible. There is also the cost of the craft materials to consider.

There is no limit to the mindful activities that you can do. If you don't think of yourself as a creative or crafty person, ask friends who are to give you simple ideas that you can share. You could also go to a craft shop and ask staff for ideas or have a browse of Pinterest. This chapter contains several examples of crafts and activities to spark your own ideas.

Knitting and needlework

When Tessa first started her women's circle, there was an invitation to bring your own crafts, and some would bring their knitting or crocheting. Tessa herself has sat doing sewing as a participant in circles and others are always fascinated to know what is being created. It's very soothing to have something repetitive to do with your hands, your eyes on what you're making and your ears open to what's being talked about. You can make the circle format spacious enough for those that know how to knit, crochet or embroider to teach those that don't and would like to learn.

Simple sewing is another activity that can be done while talking. Tessa created vulva heart decorations for fun one Christmas and has used these in circles where the topic was pelvic health. The decorations can be sewn in 70 minutes using pre-cut felt shapes. People can choose from different colours of felt, ribbon and thread to make their own unique craft. Instructions for this decoration can be found through Tessa's website (see www. tessavenutisanderson.co.uk/menstrual-cycle-awareness/resources).

The Red Dress is a project conceived by British artist Kirstie Macleod (see https://reddressembroidery.com). She had women around the world embroider designs to contribute to a single incredible dress. Where a circle is meeting over a longer period of time, a larger collaborative project could be undertaken like a quilt or wall hanging.

Connecting crafts with the circle process/topic

Making something relevant to the circle process or topic can bring the subject alive. When Julia created a 'new moon' circle in her studio, the first activity was to decorate the listening stick that was used at each gathering. Each person had the opportunity to add colourful material to the stick. This activity also brought into the circle the idea of each person deciding to pick up the stick when they felt moved to speak and to place it back in the centre of the circle when they had finished. The co-creation of the stick helped add to the importance of the rule of circle not to interrupt someone while they held the stick.

In mother and daughter circles, Tessa brought air-drying clay to create figurines to represent the feminine. The mums were asked to bring a chopping board to model the clay on and different implements were shared to make marks on the clay. It was made clear that it was about getting your hands dirty and having fun, rather than creating a masterpiece. Talking continued about what it meant to be female today, and after everyone had finished making their item (which were not only figurines but also bowls and 3D pictures), they explained the meaning of each one.

In girls' and women's circles, Tessa has also brought the materials to make bracelets that represent the menstrual cycle, with different coloured beads to represent different phases. This facilitates learning as the number of beads used and the length of the bracelets represent different length cycles. For these activities, it's useful to have a couple of examples ready made that can be passed around.

Sometimes the subject of the circle lends itself to a particular activity. In one circle, Julia introduced the topic of 'How we see ourselves and how we perceive other people see us'. Each person participating was invited to create a self-portrait: not to look like them but to give an idea of who they were. It was a fun activity that required no painting ability.

Julia also used creating self-portraits to bring alive the topic of 'Start before you are ready'. This was a reflection of the belief that men often apply for jobs that they do not yet have the qualifications for but believe they can achieve, whereas women often wait until they are overqualified before feeling confident enough to apply. Creating a self-portrait facilitated discussions around how we see ourselves and what we can do to become more confident to try new activities and apply for roles that might be a stretch. Collage with images from magazines can be another way of supporting people who consider themselves less artistic to join in.

Co-creating bunting is another collective activity that can be fun if you have an event coming up. Triangles made of material will make the longest-lasting bunting, but paper/card and ribbon can work beautifully too.

Planting seeds can be a particularly fun activity with children. If creating a circle that lasts a number of weeks, you could plant something at the start that grows throughout the time. If you decide to do this, then it is helpful to decide where the plant might be stored between weeks. Some people may not be able to store plants easily or remember to water them.

Planting seeds can be symbolic of the journey that you're on together, the connection and care between you.

As you can see, there are so many ways that you can support the talking and listening element through crafts.

Mindful colouring

Mindful colouring is something that can keep eyes and hands busy, while talking happens. Etsy is a great source of colouring images on different themes that can be downloaded and printed. Another way is to purchase a colouring book connected to the theme of your circle, cut the pages out of the book and invite people to choose one to colour in. Ask in advance that attendees bring felt-tip pens or colouring pencils and something to lean on if you're not around a table.

Co-created centrepiece

Creating a centrepiece can happen while the circle is under way. As a facilitator, you can provide material as a base and the items to create the centrepiece, or ask people to bring items with them. A symmetrical mandala is a very satisfying activity to co-create. Leaves and flowers can be collected for the purpose, or bowls of lentils, dried beans and rice can provide an attractive array of colours.

It's easier to make a symmetrical design if you mark out quarters on your base in advance with ribbon or one of the items (rice in a line works well). Then you invite a couple of participants at a time to make the same design in each of the quadrants, moving around the material.

Journalling

Journalling is a more solitary activity but can support reflective time before sharing in the bigger circle. When journalling (see the section 'Exploring through journalling' in Chapter 9 for prompts), some people in your circle may feel more comfortable drawing pictures. With any writing activity, it can therefore be helpful to bring coloured pens and give the option of drawing or doodling.

After journalling, it is important to reconnect with the circle by inviting people to share what came up (content) or how it felt to give space to this topic (process). If the content of what someone has written or drawn is too private, talking about the process instead can enable sharing.

Activity-focused circle

Sometimes due to the demographic or topic, the activity is the focus while the talking and listening happen more informally around it. The Frome Men's Shed is an example of crafting and fixing enabling talking, although in a less formal way than a talking circle.

At the family Santosa yoga camp, fire making was a popular activity with the children. All sorts of wonderful conversations about growing up happened around that activity while everyone was busy creating a fire from scratch.

With certain activities, like woodwork, their nature may determine the venue and what the space looks like – for example, workbenches side by side rather than a circular format.

EXERCISE: LET'S GET CREATIVE

Read this through and then close your eyes to head down memory lane.

When you were a small child, with no conceptions of whether an activity was useful or not, or the outcome of an activity was considered 'good' or not, what did you enjoy?

Perhaps it was at home, at school, at a playgroup, or outside with other kids.

Was there anything that could absorb you for hours?

Were there activities that involved using your hands?

Julia and Tessa remember making potions from petals in jars of water, cutting up magazines to make collages, embroidering little pictures from embroidery sets while watching TV, spending hours knitting a jumper and drawing still life.

Of course, not all circles are talking ones. You might have a circle celebrating the equinoxes or solstices and invite people to share something, such as poems, music or songs, or lead a little meditation. In this way, you provide a collective experience rather than talking about experiences.

Activities which mark beginnings and endings can be powerful. An activity could include writing down something that people would like to be released and then burning it to indicate completion, or writing wishes and then using the ritual of burning to send the wishes out into the world. If deciding to utilise fire, then safety regulations need to be considered. These activities work particularly well for:

- end-of-year and New Year circles

- summer solstice circle (because the solstice is the beginning of days shortening)

- end of a series of circles, retreat or training

- a circle focused on transformation

- mother blessings or menopause celebrations

- puberty rites of passage.

If you have access to a river, lake or the sea, you could create a ceremony of letting go. Ask people to bring a natural object that can float on water and use it to symbolise what they are letting go of. Providing seeds or seedlings to take away and sow/plant could end a gathering on a hopeful note.

Singing and music

As we talked about in Chapter 11, singing and music can be an effective way of uniting people and creating atmosphere. Care does need to be taken when music becomes part of an activity as some people enjoy singing and making music far more than others. If craft and music are brought together, those people less inclined to sing can feel involved by taking part in the craft aspect of the activity.

Creating something while singing is an activity that can be used to bond a group. It is as if you are charging up the objects being made with a special energy. For example, bracelets can be made, using the same sort of thread for each one and a selection of beads to choose from or a number of threads that are plaited. The bracelet becomes a memento of the gathering for every participant. No special knowledge of how to create a bracelet is necessary and the time required for creation is short.

We encourage you to be inventive with your creativity and also be very clear about the purpose of any activity or craft. Is it being used to serve the purpose of your gathering or is it a 'keeping the hands busy' activity that facilitates tricky conversations? Maybe it is most successful when the two are combined.

CIRCLE STORY: BECOMING MUMS AND THE MOTHERS' QUILT

Fi McQuay and Beth Allum are the co-founders of Becoming Mums, based in Reading, Berkshire. They got fed up with talking about nappies and wanted to create a space where mums could connect with others and find people who 'got it'. They identified a feeling of isolation that can happen even when attending a busy playgroup and wanted to create a different kind of space where people can talk honestly.

Along with peer-to-peer support sessions with facilitated themed conversations, led by the group themselves, they run creative projects. One project that they did in partnership with textile artist Kate Powell involved creating a collaborative quilt that celebrated all the ways in which mothers are queens and the qualities that both roles require, such as leadership, love, strength and courage. The quilt was made over a number of workshops around Reading and at WaterFest with scraps of fabric from many different people's parenting journeys.

Funding came from Reading Borough Council and the Arts Council. Mothers from local schools who might most benefit were identified by involved schools' family support workers. The completed quilt travelled to Reading Minster, a church in Central Reading, for the commemoration service for her Majesty the Queen. It has created a sense of pride for those who contributed, and in the process much honest talk helped people feel less alone in parenting.

Many of us who do not regularly take part in activities like painting, drawing, writing or arts and crafts may not view ourselves as creative.

When we introduce arts and crafts to a circle gathering, it is important to make it clear that there is no need for people to create something that is of a particular standard. In UK schools, children from a very young age are graded on their creativity and judge themselves and their creative ability. Circle is a perfect opportunity to debunk this myth and free up our participants to create for creativity's sake.

CIRCLE STORY: TEEN CIRCLE

Cecilia was given the opportunity to take over a teen yoga circle. It was a group of girls between the ages of 10 and 16. The room was large enough for it to be easy to gather in a circle. She decided to introduce craft to the circle in the first week as an easy way to learn a little more about the girls she was supporting. The first activity was to create seasonal dials that represented the seasonal and lunar cycles.

Cecilia gently introduced the topic of the menstrual cycle and would bring a craft into each session so that the girls could do something simple with their hands and be less self-conscious about what they were talking about.

She noticed as the weeks went on that the girls were much less interested in the physical aspects of yoga and wanted to rest and talk. Slowly, the girls began to open up about their experience with their menstrual cycle, their feelings around gender and their choices around pronouns.

Although the circle had moved away from yoga and movement, Cecilia decided not to change the name of the circle. In order to respect the needs of the girls and the discussions that emerged around the menstrual cycle, she kept the group female. For parents of boys who wished to attend, she signposted other teen yoga classes.

If someone joins your circle and they have been given no advance warning that craft will be part of the session, they might feel uncomfortable. They might believe they are not a talented enough artist to draw or paint or create arts and crafts. The idea of doing crafts can bring up fear and memories of school for people who were told they were not good enough. The next exercise can support someone to explore crafts from a new perspective and enjoy crafts for their own sake.

● EXERCISE: CREATIVITY CIRCLE

This activity could be introduced with a poem about bravery, courage, making mistakes, taking a first step – something that connects to the theme of creativity.

The participants could be invited to close their eyes and imagine something they are creating or would like to create.

They could then be invited to write or draw freely around the subject.

Each person could be invited to share their response to the poem should they choose to, either directly speaking to what they are creating or indirectly as to whether the activity helped with their process.

This activity is particularly helpful if there is a specific project those taking part are working towards. If this is expressed specifically as a theme for the circle, then it is more likely that those attending will come along with the intention of working on a particular creative endeavour.

There are many examples of circles where activity causes people to find it easier to speak. When activities are taking place, there is less need for eye contact, so someone who feels shy or vulnerable may be more likely to speak.

CIRCLE STORY: INTRODUCING RITUAL
Tessa shares:

> A memorable experience was a sleepover we'd arranged to extend the women's circle over a weekend. On Sunday, after breakfast, we gathered around a fire pit in the woods. I had made a simple felt doll to symbolise the 'good girl', 'good daughter', 'good wife' or 'good mother' that we might sense in ourselves.
>
> We sat round the fire talking about how 'being good' limited us. I then put on some music with strong drumming in it and people played drums and percussion instruments around the fire. Some people got up to dance.
>
> There was a sense of freedom after spending the weekend talking honestly with each other. You could feel people letting go of worrying about what others thought about them. I got out the felt doll and invited people to project all the limiting 'good' behaviours onto the doll and then threw her in the fire!
>
> I thought she would burn very quickly. Instead, she slowly curled up and blackened. Eventually, she was consumed by the fire and it seemed like everyone was holding their breath for the duration of that process. Would those limiting 'good' behaviours really be allowed to go? It was a very powerful moment that I know stayed with the women.

Introducing ritual and ceremony to circle time can add potency to the transformation that happens. If you're interested in developing this aspect of circle time, visit others' circles where this happens to observe how it makes you feel and what makes it stand out.

As you think about the possibilities of complementary activities, return to your intention for the circle. Will the activity facilitate talking and listening? Have you included the cost of materials in the price of the circle or asked people to bring their own materials? How can you make it accessible for everyone?

In the next chapter, we focus on circles for children, as there are different considerations. And lots of fun to be had!

CHAPTER 14

Children, Teens and Talking Circles

The children come into the space, some bouncing in, others cautious. They see intriguing things laid out around the centrepiece and want to know about them immediately. Settling in with a quick icebreaker of easy questions, they're ready to be involved. Flowing between different activities to get them moving and ones to get them interested in the topic and listening, the time flies by.

A talking circle with children feels different to one with adults. The pace of the activities is much quicker and the event would usually be shorter. Activities are often the key to a successful children's circle.

When circle time is experienced at a young age, the relationships founded on deep listening can last a lifetime and the model of communicating respectfully is taken into adulthood.

I am such a hater of PSHE [personal, social, health and economic education classes]. It is the biggest waste of time. It is taught in a classroom. Everywhere I have been, the teacher stands at the front, they talk about something that needs to be discussed, like abortion or drugs or self-harm, and then you fill in this worksheet. You do not learn anything.

It would be a much more valuable experience to have a conversation about what happened and what went wrong and add something... Instead of everyone just sitting there or leaving the classroom crying because they are so triggered, and no-one really learns anything. Schools should have more places to hold circles. The standard of education would be better if we learnt that way.

Anouska (teen)

Let's start with some examples of circles for children and teens to get your imagination going:

- Co-creating a story with a focus on how to manage big emotions.

- Parent and pre-teen daughter circle focusing on changing bodies and periods.

- Teen yoga with circle check-in.

- Circle about the environment with crafts using natural materials.

- Circle in the woods with talking while learning fire-lighting and whittling.

- Home education circle with educational games.

- Teen circle without adults for discussion of relationships and social media.

What you'll notice is usually it is not only talking that happens, but other activities are involved, whether it's crafts, yoga or learning new skills. Refer to the example 'Mother and daughter circles' circle in Chapter 9 for the variety of activities included in one event.

Obviously, the activity and topic need to be age-appropriate. With preschoolers, circle time can be modelled by the parents talking while the children have activities to do connected with the topic. For kids in infant school (5–8 years), creating a story together around the topic is a good way to engage and share ideas. The amount of talking you expect from the children can increase as they get older, with teen circles without adults facilitating being possible if they have experienced circle time before or have the right guidance beforehand.

Supporting talking in children's circles

Icebreakers can be used for a fun and simple way to get over any reticence to talk. You can invite people to ask the person next to them (or their parent) what their favourite dessert is and then share it with the group. Or beforehand, you might have asked them to bring something special to share with the circle, perhaps something relevant to the event's topic. If they're old enough to write, you can ask them to write down a word or draw a picture for how they feel at the beginning of the group and acknowledge that different feelings, including shyness, are normal.

Just as in an adult talking circle, guidelines can be outlined in an age-appropriate way. Partly, this may be to help them realise that this is a different space from school. You can say that if people talk over each other, you can't concentrate or hear everyone that wants to share, and so if people do, they'll hear this sound (e.g. a drum, chime, horn) and remember to talk one at a time. Sitting on the floor in a circle will be more conducive to sitting behind tables as at school, and you can encourage people to bring cushions and blankets to make their own nest.

Mark Walsh shared where his passion for circle time started:

> A lot of my whole life's work is a reaction to my education experience in a state school…controlling, bullied by teachers… One or two teachers held discussions. It felt freer and more respectful. The first inkling that something else was possible.

You may decide to start the circle with activities to capture the children's attention. See the following section for ideas on colouring and mandala-making. The activity can be explained and then the structure for the rest of the time shared so that everyone can settle, knowing what to expect. While the children are engaged with a simple activity, you may find they are able to relax and be more open to the topic of the circle.

When parents are present in the circle, it is helpful for them to start off the talking and model how it is done in this setting. In talking circles about puberty, Tessa will speak to the mums or other caregivers before the event to outline the kind of experiences that are helpful to share. This provides time to reflect on what would be constructive for the girls to hear. Perhaps where mums had a difficult time with periods, a different aspect of puberty can be chosen to talk about. The variety of experiences that are heard from different people are so helpful to the children. Bella (10 years old), who attended such an event, said, 'Before I came [to the event] I felt nervous. I didn't know what to expect. But then I liked learning about puberty with my mum. I made new friends and would like to do this again.'

Props and activities to support talking

In general, providing some props to support talking is helpful. For example, having key words connected to the theme written out in big letters and selecting pictures connected to the topic can spark ideas. Another example is to read out a story or poem to illustrate the theme. *Little Mouse and the Red Wall* by Britta Teckentrup (2018) is a favourite, with beautiful illustrations talking about emotions and being brave. With smaller children, having puppets or soft toys could make communicating the topic fun and accessible.

For supporting children to express emotions, picture cards can be used to make it easier for them to work out how they feel by giving suggestions. You can make your own or purchase existing ones such as 'Bear cards' or 'Strength cards' (available from https://innovativeresources. org/resources). Bear cards have illustrations of bears feeling different emotions. There are no words and it's up to the viewer to decide what a particular drawing of a bear is expressing. Strength cards have a picture and a word, so children need to be able to read them to select the quality they want to express, such as 'friendly' or 'enthusiastic'.

Big emotions can emerge even with the most neutral topics. Refer to Chapter 10 on circle dynamics and consider choosing a venue where it's possible to find a quiet space if a child has become overwhelmed. For younger children, inviting them to bring a special toy and a familiar blanket to make a cosy space can provide a source of comfort. The parent will know what comforts the child, but it's important to create a space where everyone knows that it's okay for emotions to be shown. You might say, 'I sometimes feel [sad, overwhelmed, angry] and after I've told someone and said how I feel, I usually feel much better.'

Including activities while talking can help take the spotlight off the person who is currently speaking. Colouring in can be a wonderful way to mindfully occupy children so that even those who are less confident artistically can be involved. A mindful activity can mean the chitter chatter of the mind is quietened and the children are more able to hear what someone is saying.

Creating a mandala out of objects you provide or natural objects that the circle participants bring to the gathering can be another way of being creative and co-producing something. Children can also be supported to sew simple items like a felt locket, bookmarks or decorations. Be aware that not all of the adults will have the skills to sew, so it's important to show everyone an example of what you're making and how to make it.

Tessa runs groups with girls aged 7–12 and finds that activities such as applying henna to the back of a hand or a foot is really popular (with consideration about how schools might respond to visible henna). Another popular activity is decorating their faces with biodegradable glitter (with a sticky cream/moisturiser to attach it).

If you have outside space, learning how to build a fire is always popular as an activity, or making popcorn or pizza on an outside fire. Popcorn can be made with two metal sieves wired together and attached to a long stick. For pizza, a simple dough can be made beforehand and cooked in a frying pan over the fire for two minutes each side, and then ingredients can be added to the top by the children. Talking can happen while the children take turns to cook their food.

Also popular around a fire is to write notes (e.g. aspirations) on paper, or 'flash paper' that burns as if by magic in a flash, to throw onto the fire. With any writing activity for children, it is helpful to check beforehand with parents if any of them have learning differences that may affect their writing ability so that alternatives can be found without embarrassment for the child.

It is well worth looking at pre-established organisations when considering working with children. There is much we can learn from organisations like the Scouts movement about how to give children the space to feel autonomous, and often these include learning new skills or enjoying craft activities.

Using movement in children's circles

Having movement breaks is another way to keep kids' engagement through the event. This can be done through games such as 'Laugh like [a duck, your mum, Father Christmas (if appropriate for your demographic)...]'. Invite people to stand up. You as the facilitator give the instruction and everyone at the same time pretends to laugh in the way that a duck, their mum or anything else you can think of would laugh, with actions like flapping wings or clutching their belly. The laughter will become real!

Another idea is copying the slow movements of a partner. Model what you mean by facing someone (seated or standing), both of you facing your palms forwards, but without touching the other person's (so it's not too easy to keep up). One person is in charge, slowly moving their hands in different shapes, with the other person copying. After a while, swap over so the other person can have a chance to lead. Keep an eye on whether the movements are getting too quick to follow, and if so, give a reminder to slow down. Putting on some calming music can support this.

Usually up to the age of about ten, we've found that children are generally comfortable with dancing in a group like this. Putting on some music for 3–5 minutes and showing some simple dance moves is a great way to break up the talking and use some energy. For older children, this activity would be easier to include in a regular circle where they have had a chance to get to know each other first.

If you are trained in yoga, leading five minutes of partner yoga with parent and child paired, or children paired, can provide a break from the talking element and get people moving. Even if you are not a yoga teacher, a simple activity you can include is to invite everyone to come into tree pose with one foot against the other leg and arms out to the side for balance. This can be done in a circle to create a wood, with fingertips touching those of their neighbours, and moving arms for swaying branches. Where they have come with a parent, if you know someone in the group wouldn't be comfortable with touching hands with strangers, you can do this activity in pairs facing each other.

To close the circle, reading a story while snuggling with a parent is an activity that can provide some relaxation and reflection time, and much appreciated bonding with children. We recommend having cushions and blankets to get cosy. This can be used towards the end of a circle to allow time for integration and some quiet time if the activities have become boisterous or the topic has been a sensitive one. Tessa has found that in the Celebration Day for Girls (usually 10- to 12-year-olds), tweens still love a cuddle with Mum.

For older children, finishing with a one- or two-word check-in can be enough. Another way to check in is to ask everyone at the same time to raise their hands and give either a thumbs-up gesture for feeling good, thumbs pointing to each other for neutral or okay, and thumbs down for feeling bad. This gives you a chance to see how the circle has been experienced and offer support or signposting where needed (e.g. to the school nurse).

Special considerations for children's circles

Below we consider some of the different factors that you might want to consider when planning your circle with children, such as age, special needs and so on. Before any session with children, be clear about the age group you will be working with and whether it will support your intention to mix different ages of children. Mixing age groups can be incredibly positive, with older children gaining a sense of pride in guiding younger ones and younger children's confidence increasing by being noticed by the older ones.

Israh Goodall shares from her own experience:

For the younger girls, it provided a space to listen to the older girls and hear what they were facing. So much of what was being spoken about were real-life challenges and questions that they too will likely be facing soon. It was very moving to see what happened as the girls began to ask each other questions and deeply listen to each other. We would be sitting and talking about our bodies or cycles or what power means, and they would be hearing it from their peers rather than from an adult. When held respectfully, this certainly feels like one of the best forms of education.

The younger girls in the group also provided an incredible gift to the older ones. Often the younger girls had a far greater ease with play, eager to roll around, play games and giggle. So often as we get older into our later teens, this changes, and there is often a real block for people to allow themselves to play in this way. It was fantastic to see the playfulness and the light-heartedness of the younger girl calling those same qualities into the older teenager.

It is helpful to either have a quick phone call with parents or create a questionnaire for parents beforehand where you can ask about specific needs and differences and what they find useful with regard to supporting the children. We have not experienced issues where there is a disagreement between the facilitator and the parent during a circle. Taking the time before an event to check in with a parent, to explain briefly how the gathering will work and what will be covered, helps manage expectations on content and behaviour.

While training may be required for certain differences in children, it is very likely that your circle can be more inclusive by asking the parents about specific needs. If this is done before the circle, then any difference can be accommodated for the whole group without singling out any child with a specific need. Circle time is a great opportunity to be inclusive in ways that may not have been available to children in other extracurricular environments where a level of proficiency in the activity may be required.

For children with sensory needs, it may be important to consider how overwhelming an environment may be and offer a separate quiet place. Shorter sessions might to easier to engage with, and there may be particular triggers for dysregulation that you can adapt for through discussion with the parent. They may want to be there to listen and not have the focus directed to them, so you will need to work together to make it a positive experience.

There are organisations that have been specifically designed to support particular needs for young children and teens, such as Teenage Cancer Trust and Grief Encounters. There are also organisations that have been formed to create better education for PSHE (personal, social, health and economic education) – for example, the work of Dr Sophie King-Hill. Having an understanding of how talking and listening circles can work for children can help you make a more informed decision as to whether to become involved with a pre-existing organisation or whether to go about your own work.

Some examples we have given have arisen out of gaps where maybe PSHE in school has not fulfilled the needs of the children. Listening circles for children do not need to be complicated and can make a huge difference in their development and reduce feelings of isolation and loneliness. Lee Keylock, who works in schools, says, 'There is not a teenager on the planet that doesn't want to be seen and heard. Even the most introverted kids want to feel validated in their lives.'

● EXERCISE: PLANNING YOUR CHILDREN'S CIRCLE

Have a pen and paper ready. There are lots of questions here and you don't need to answer them all in one sitting. Write down your answers or create a mind map to support your reflection.

Who is it for?

- Who is your circle for?

- What age range are you looking to work with?

- Would you like a multigenerational aspect to your circle?

- Will the circle be for every child or a specific demographic?

- Are you planning to run the circle for parents and children?

What is the aim of the circle?

- What is your circle for? Write or draw your reasons for holding the event.

- Is this need being met anywhere else in your community? (If so, could you join forces or share facilities?)

- Will the circle be educational? (If so, how will you make it fun? How will this differ from their experience in formal education settings?)

Structure of your circle

- How long will the circle be? (Research what works for those that already work with this age group.)

- Do you have time constraints or a specific time frame you have to work with? (e.g. lunch break or after school club?)

- Will this be a series or one-off circle? (e.g. for a term or the end of the school year?)

Logistics of circle

- Have you considered the location for your circle and its suitability for activities? (Especially if they involve cooking or the potential for mess or damage, e.g. henna staining.)

- Is outside activity possible and do you have a contingency plan for wet weather?

- Do you have the required consent forms for any activities and insurance to cover them?

- Do you want to provide refreshments/have the facilities to do so? (If so, are you aware of allergies?)

- What support do you need in place for safeguarding? (See the section 'Safeguarding in children's circles' at the end of this chapter.)

Activities to support the talking

- How can you keep the children engaged in the topic through movement or other activities?

- Do you have skills in movement practices and/or arts and crafts that could be used with children?

- Will parents have to supply any materials for the event?

Marketing and admin

- Is the circle a commercial venture, a free community space, a collaboration with school or place of worship? (If in collaboration, have you shared in writing how you will communicate, share that the event is happening, and be paid if appropriate?)

- How can you promote your circle?

- What will you charge for the circle? (If you're volunteering your time, do you need a minimal charge for any craft material costs?)

Dream into making a fun and informative session. With the topic in mind, what related games, movement, fun activities, crafts and/or refreshments can you include?

Now put all of that to one side and go back to your intention for running the session. Connect with the need that you have identified and sit with that.

Often, people are called to run circles with children because they want to give them a different experience from what is available in the mainstream education system.

CIRCLE STORY: COMPLEMENTING THE SCHOOL CURRICULUM

Knowing that Tessa ran menstrual cycle awareness workshops for adults, a couple of mums approached her at her daughters' primary school to ask if she would run a session for their girls. Relationship and sex education (RSE) always seems to happen right at the end of the summer term, or at least the part that makes the children giggly, and they felt that there was so much more they wanted their girls to know.

The curriculum covers the absolute basics in primary school, but since 10 per cent of girls will start their period while in Key Stage 2, it would be helpful if they were taught more. Tessa created a two-hour session for 7–9-year-olds that focused on how bodies begin to change, a simple way of charting (starting with emotions), the concept of the inner seasons (a season for each of the four phases of the menstrual cycle) and an introduction to all the period products that are available. This event was held in a local yoga studio and mums attended with their daughters. A key part was hearing the mums talk about their own experience of their bodies changing.

She has also run talks at schools for the parents on how to talk to your kids about their changing bodies. It would be wonderful to do this in a circle format, but attending a talk on this topic challenges some people a lot. Tessa has always asked the schools to communicate that it is for parents of any age child, but the majority have children in Year 5 and 6 because that's when they see their own or others' kids starting to change. Having a contact to introduce you to the school is key.

From these experiences, Tessa wrote a book called *Ruby Luna's Curious Journey* for kids five years old and upwards. The sooner parents answer questions about bodies, the easier it is for everyone. Amazing creative projects can come out of talking circles when you can see there is a need that is not being met!

Safeguarding in children's circles

There is responsibility that comes with running events for children. If you are alone with the children, it would be wise to obtain a Disclosure and Barring Service (DBS) check if you are in the UK. This can be obtained through the UK government website and gives parents a level of reassurance. Please check with your country what safeguarding requirements there are for working with children and young adults.

Developing a policy around duty of care will help you be clear what are your responsibilities to report child protection or welfare concerns to children's services or the police. In a talking circle, a child may experience a higher level of connection or trust than they usually have with an adult and disclose something. The Early Years Alliance provides information on how to create policies and procedures.

The next chapter addresses challenges in circles, some of which may be a red flag to those attending. Having looked at best practice, it's useful to look from a different perspective.

CHAPTER 15

Challenges in Circles

You're sitting in a group in a circle setting and something feels off. You can't put your finger on it, but you know that you don't feel comfortable to share much beyond your name. You can feel yourself biding time until it would be polite to leave. Afterwards, there's a feeling of disappointment that you didn't get that sense of connection you were hoping for.

Whether it's in a formal talking circle or another group dynamic, you probably have had the experience of not feeling that you fit in and not being comfortable to fully share. In this chapter, we want to outline the challenges in a circle context to validate these types of experiences and to support your reflection on your own facilitation. Let's remember that we're human and sometimes have an off-day: this chapter is not about running circles perfectly all of the time, but creating as strong a container as we can for the benefit of all participants!

We reflected long and hard on whether to include this chapter because the aim of the book is to provide a positive guide to facilitating listening and talking circles. However, it is important to validate people's negative experiences of circle time. We hope that including these challenges provides a different perspective to look at what is and isn't good practice.

It might be that the guidelines for how the gathering works have not been clear and so you're confused about how to behave and what is expected. Perhaps you feel like the odd one out and therefore guarded. Maybe the facilitator has let someone dominate with a rant or allowed people to talk over each other and the space doesn't feel held in the way you would like. Maybe the activity or craft introduced feels too difficult or you are being asked to participate in an unexpected way that feels too uncomfortable. There are key issues that can be seen as 'red flags' that are worth being aware of both as a facilitator and a participant in talking circles.

We can learn as much from what can go wrong as what it looks like when it goes right. We have divided these factors into the themes of power dynamics, organisation, facilitation of circle, quality of communication and expectations.

Power dynamics

There are different ways power dynamics play out in talking circles:

- discounting expertise (formal or lived experience) of attendees
- not acknowledging the power imbalance if there is one (e.g. with children)
- facilitator assuming too much authority (e.g. guru complex)
- anarchistic circle with no clear leadership or facilitator being responsible
- not taking responsibility for the circle (e.g. with follow-up support)
- absence of diversity, which can evoke feelings of discomfort for those in the minority
- putting self or others in a position of being a fixer or healer.

The purpose of a circle is to minimise power dynamics and provide a space for equal sharing. This is easy to say, but requires self-reflection from the facilitator, clear description about who the circle is for and guidance about how communication works in a circle situation. Returning to the intention for the circle (see Chapter 3) can clarify what the motivation is behind a gathering: who and what is it for?

Tanya Forgan shared, 'There were no spaces for me to go because the circles I went to were mainly white women. So for me to bring that piece of work did not feel safe' (talking about the need to create circles for people of dual heritage). Sometimes the challenge experienced in a circle space leads to an intention to meet a need that is not being met.

Organisation of gatherings

How a circle is organised can create issues:

- not outlining guidelines for the circle (e.g. resulting in allowing people to come and go as they wish, which is not helpful in most events; confidentiality breaches)

- lack of structure (e.g. resulting in boredom, confusion, anxiety)

- facilitator not being sufficiently prepared

- running over time

- unpaid circles potentially resulting in burnout for the organiser

- not creating a space that is suitable for the gathering (e.g. no toilets, overlooked).

When a circle is run well, it seems effortless and easy to do. However, a lot of preparation goes into creating a successful event with a strong container for the sharing. From setting up the space and settling yourself (Chapter 5) and laying out the guidelines (Chapter 8), to spending time on creating a schedule for the circle, with what happens when and the approximate timings, is essential (Chapter 9). If you are not naturally a good timekeeper, ask an attendee at the circle who is to keep an eye on time for you and let you know when it is time for closing.

Holding/facilitation of circle time

The circle dynamics can be affected by the skill of facilitation. Poor facilitation can lead to a number of problems:

- Having no boundaries or unclear boundaries for the setting

- Thinking that you know better than someone else how deep they can go

- Pushing people to be more involved than they would like to be

- Disproportional space taking (e.g. one person dominating the talking)

- Not responding to the needs of the participants

- Including too much teaching ('When is it a classroom and when is it a circle?').

How the circle is framed, in terms of boundaries, guidelines, precepts or whatever term resonates for you, is the foundation of good facilitation. When the sharing in the circle does not feel healthy for everyone, the container can be reset at any time by checking in with those present and re-establishing the guidelines. Refer back to Chapter 10 on circle dynamics for tips.

Lydia Martin shared from the perspective of a circle attendee:

> I remember a circle where one person spoke so vividly of their experiences and for such a long time that I felt inadequate, like I hadn't experienced enough to be valid, and unheard. I didn't feel as though I had opportunity to share. I felt as though anything I would share wouldn't be interesting.

Remember, as the facilitator it is not rude to facilitate how people are talking or how long they are talking for – it is your responsibility. You may feel like you are interrupting, but we invite you to reframe it as keeping the container a welcoming space for everyone.

Quality of communication

In everyday life, there are problems with communications that we aim to avoid in a talking and listening circle:

- shaming someone who has said something that could offend other members of the group

- solutions being given unsolicited

- people not owning what they are saying (e.g. using 'you', 'we' or 'they' instead of 'I')

- having no space for feedback or reflection after the circle.

In everyday conversation, it is common to be judged for what you say, be given solutions when you just want to share your experience and to lessen the impact of what you say by talking in general terms.

Circle attendees will fall into old habits of communication, but the role of the facilitator is to clearly state the guidelines to support respectful listening and talking, and maintain those values themselves and within the gathering. As a facilitator, you are not going to get this right all the time, but if you see recurring types of behaviour, it's a good time to address what is happening. This can be gently – for example, 'I'm reflecting on how I want to find a solution for [Name]'s issue, but s/he hasn't asked for one.' Refer to Chapter 10 on circle dynamics for tips.

Facilitator and participant expectations

In the circle, it's important to manage your expectations as a new facilitator, and those of new attendees. The following are signs that more guidance around communication is needed:

- having a specific expectation for others' experience

- thinking you need something huge to happen for the circle to have been a success

- not setting expectations around communication/etiquette for being in circle

- feeling worse after the circle on a regular basis

- you just don't feel 'right'

- makes you feel judged, shamed or emotionally exposed.

Facilitators want to provide a positive experience, and people attending want to come out feeling understood. As Kate Codrington says, 'We seldom come to a gathering where it is promoted as a dangerous badland!' We all have subconscious expectations, and it's helpful to explicitly manage expectations in your communications.

If someone in your circle experienced any of these challenges, hopefully they would feel comfortable enough to have a conversation with you as the facilitator and share their concerns. This creates a learning opportunity for you to improve the experience for others.

EXERCISE: LEARNING FROM UNCOMFORTABLE EXPERIENCES

Take a moment to read through and reflect. Then write down your thoughts, draw, or even record yourself talking about your experience. This exercise can also be used in listening partnership with another circle holder.

Remember a time when you attended a circle or other group experience where you felt uncomfortable. Can you pinpoint what made you uncomfortable? Whose (if anyone's) responsibility was it to create a container where you felt safe and able to share? Can you re-imagine the experience so that someone stepped in to make it okay or put guidelines in place to prevent the discomfort?

As a facilitator, what can you take away from the experience about how you will do things differently? How does this link to your values?

Are there other challenges in circle spaces that weren't identified in this chapter? What are they?

● EXERCISE: IDENTIFYING CHALLENGES IN CIRCLES

You're invited to a circle and the facilitator invites sharing to start. Although the circle was set for 60 minutes, one person took up over 20 minutes with their share, leaving little time for other people.

The facilitator said after 30 minutes of the gathering that she'd forgotten to talk about confidentiality. The number of people invited to this online circle was unlimited so there was not space for everyone to participate, and a couple of people joined 40 minutes in.

It felt as though you were invited solely as witnesses rather than participants, and although everyone was invited to share, it was clear that there was not sufficient time for equal sharing to occur.

Can you identify the challenges in this event? What action would you take next time if you were the facilitator to make it a better experience for everyone? What would your schedule for timings and checklist of things to cover look like?

Asking for feedback from participants about what it's like to be in the circle might feel daunting but can be a brilliant way of checking how the container is functioning. You might also reflect on who attends the event, and if there is regularly a demographic missing that you wanted to attract, why that might be. Having supervision with someone qualified or a listening partnership with another facilitator could be useful for reflective practice.

We hope that this chapter has given you lots of food for thought rather than making holding a circle a daunting prospect. It provides a different perspective on the previous content in the book and hopefully enables you to hold up a mirror to your facilitation and become an even better, humble circle holder.

In the next chapter, we explore facilitating online talking and listening circles, which can have their own challenges and benefits.

CHAPTER 16

Online Gatherings

You want to connect with others beyond the local area and connect from the comfort of your own home. You set up a space to join the circle, light a candle, get a drink and log in through your device. A whole world opens up: different from an in-person circle and enabling connection from afar or on a niche topic. Your facilitation is just as important in an online circle.

Beautiful connections can be formed between people and tender experiences shared online. People can gather from a far wider geographical location, lending depth and breadth to the experience. There are no travel challenges and people who may otherwise be unable to attend circle due to cost, logistics, family or work responsibilities, or physical or energy challenges can attend. In lockdown, many people who had been excluded from gathering in groups, including those with chronic health conditions and mobility issues, were able to meet with others.

In our yoga communities, this was most successful for isolated older members, who flocked to online classes and mastered the technology far quicker than they expected. All these factors make online circles more accessible than in-person options for many. There are minimal costs for participants and the risks are also far lower for the circle holder.

> I enjoy the palpable energy of being in person, but online for me, the online shift reconnected me with people who I may have lost due to distance. It is beautiful for connecting people from all over the world. The accessibility that online affords us is not to be dismissed. As a lone parent, if more things had been online as my daughter was growing up, I think I would have felt less isolated.

There are some people who are more free in an online situation to address their own needs. They are more likely to choose what suits them best when they are in their own space.

Cecilia Allon

For some people, their nervous systems can relax when they join a circle online and they are more comfortable making connections that way than in person.

Some circles are created with very specific groups in mind who are unlikely to be able to meet easily in person. The online option allows for a far wider group to gather. For example, the charity Support after Murder and Manslaughter (SAMM) offers opportunities for people affected to attend meetings online so that support is available at the click of a Zoom link on a weekly basis. The logistics involved in creating such a gathering in person would be huge. Another advantage of online gathering is that if someone is hard of hearing, finds it difficult to follow speech or does not have the language spoken in the group as their mother tongue, captions can be enabled so that they can read what is being said and join in more comfortably.

Facilitating an online circle has similarities to in-person events and some differences. We have a lot of experience facilitating online because this is how we run many of our training courses, and so in this chapter we share some tips for making a virtual event run smoothly.

Managing who attends and how

We run our online circles through the app Zoom. A meeting can be created with a unique link to share with people who book for the circle. Enabling the Waiting Room function and having password access are safety features to prevent people attending who are not there for its intended purpose. There is also a registration function so that you capture people's names and email addresses, and can add custom questions to collect information before the event begins.

During the pandemic, the drama school that Tessa's daughters attended posted a Zoom link on a Facebook page inviting people to attend an open dance session. After the session had been going for ten minutes, a man joined who flashed the children, because there were no waiting room, passwords or other safety measures. As facilitators, it's our responsibility to safeguard against such situations where we can.

Just as with in-person circles, guidelines need to be shared to support communication in online gatherings. However, there may be some additional guidance around the technology. Some online circles require the participants to have their video on while others give space for anonymity. It depends on the nature and purpose of your circle whether participation has to be with video on. With confidential circles, it is important to know who is present, so if you decide to allow people to participate without their video on, it is recommended that you have procedures in place to ensure you know who will be present.

For example, Daniel Groom, co-founder of Queer Wellbeing, says, 'The rules for online circles are that when they arrive they have to show their face and we know everyone who gets access to the link to attend the group, to ensure safeguarding.' In contrast, the charity Support after Murder and Manslaughter (SAMM) allows for attendance in their circle without video; however, their vetting procedure before someone is welcomed into their circles ensures the circle holders are aware of who is attending and how vulnerable they may be. As facilitator, you will need to make a decision about what is right for your community.

It is helpful to send an email with guidance on what the etiquette is for attending an online circle. For example, you may encourage people to have their video on, but stay on mute unless they are currently talking. Although it may seem counter to the ethos of a talking circle to ask people to mute themselves when not speaking, it's for the functional reason that otherwise there can be disruptive background noise, an echo or disruption to the voice of the person who is speaking.

The mute function is also really valuable in that it is not possible to interrupt without unmuting yourself. Therefore, if you have a rule of not speaking over people and someone feels moved to interrupt, they are far less likely to do so because they would notice themselves moving to unmute and then realise what they have done and be more likely to respect the rule of non-interruption.

You may also ask that participants be in a private space without others listening in, because just as in an in-person circle, you don't want to be overlooked or overheard by others who aren't part of the circle.

See the template below for a confirmation email after someone has booked.

Template: Email for online circle

Dear [Name]

I am looking forward to welcoming you to:

NAME OF CIRCLE

DATE and TIME OF CIRCLE [be clear about different time zones if international]

This is a place for you to be seen, held and heard.

The purpose of the circle is to: ....

By attending, you will [list benefits connected to the aim of the circle]

Before we meet:

1. Check your device is fully charged or plugged in and that you have a good internet connection.

2. You may wish to use headphones to block out any external noises.

3. Find a private space where you and the people on the screen won't be overheard.

4. Have with you a pen and paper or something you can use for note making.

5. Have a drink to hand.

Login details: ....

Terms & Conditions [If applicable. Recommended if there is a fee to attend.]

[e.g. We do not provide refunds or exchanges for future events due to internet issues, late arrival, issues with regard to finding emails or time zone issues. Cancellations within 7 days of the event are non-refundable.]

Preparing for the circle:

[Make any suggestions here with regard to preparation – any pre-circle ritual, candle lighting and comfortable seating arrangements.]

Warmly

[YOUR NAME]

During the Covid pandemic, many people became used to receiving a recording of an event if they could not attend live. However, recording talking circles can be detrimental to creating a container. It can create a feeling of being watched and non-reciprocity. Therefore, it is important to go back to your intention for the circle and reflect on the purpose of a recording.

When you have decided whether to record the circle, it is good practice to share your intention around recording in the marketing material for the circle. If you have decided your aim is to record, you are less likely to have someone objecting if you've made it clear why and who the recording is for. Consent is essential if you are considering recording an online gathering, even when it is only being recorded for those who are present.

We do record our online training sessions, which are held in a circle format. We explain at the beginning of the training that any recording is only for the use of those participating and that all content shared by group members remains confidential.

While an online circle might seem to provide a fun photo opportunity to create a memory of the circle, you need to ask for consent before taking a screenshot or photo.

Taking turns

When a circle is online, there are two options for who talks next. One option is that as the facilitator you go around your screen and name the person to talk next, inviting them to unmute and take their turn.

The other option is what we call the 'popcorn' approach. This means that people unmute themselves when they feel ready to speak. Sometimes this results in people unmuting at the same time, but one person will usually suggest the other goes first. Sometimes on screen, it can be less easy to read the cues for when someone has finished talking and for someone else to come in. However, the circle will find its rhythm before long.

Usually in a circle, we will do a mixture of both approaches: naming the person to speak next for the initial and closing check-ins (in the order we see on our screen) and then using popcorn mode for the main sharing.

Another option is that the person currently talking chooses the next person to speak. It would be important to make it clear before you start that you can pass on to someone else if you're not ready to speak.

Similarly to an in-person circle, there may be people who tend to talk more and others who are quiet. The same strategies for including everyone can be used. Setting a time for one or two minutes and signalling when the time is up can work well. From experience, don't rely on the sound of your phone's timer to notify them as it may not be heard through your device's microphone. Instead, giving a thumbs up or other hand gesture is effective.

Listening partnerships or small group work online

Listening partnerships are a wonderful way of building connections online. Zoom has a function called 'breakout rooms' where you can divide people into different virtual meeting rooms. It is worth practising this or having the instructions printed out. You can either set an amount of time or open the rooms for an unspecified period of time.

Explain fully how listening partnerships work, the topic to talk on and how much time each person has to talk. You can send messages or broadcasts into the breakout rooms to remind people to swap over. It is also possible to drop into a breakout room to see how the activity is going, but warn people in advance if you intend to do this. After the end of the specified time, or after you have ended the time, there is 60 seconds grace and then they will automatically be brought back into the main meeting.

You can let Zoom randomly put people into rooms or manually add people if you want to put specific individuals together. It is helpful to guide people about what to do in case someone finds themselves alone in a breakout room (because the other person couldn't get in or dropped out because of internet issues): that is, return to the main room where the facilitator will be.

Once back in the main meeting room, inviting people to share their own experience of being in the listening partnership is helpful for re-establishing the feeling of being back in the circle.

Creating connection

Asking people to lean in towards the camera and look at each other can bring a feeling of intimacy as we wouldn't normally do this in a work meeting! Often the participants will start smiling at each other. This is ideal to do before the introductions start and/or at the end of the circle before you leave the meeting. You can also pair people up to gaze at each other; as Henika Patel explained, 'It was more powerful to have them looking at each other [a specific person] rather than at someone who wasn't looking back at them.'

There might usually be an element of touch in your circles, with people connecting hands on either side. Although this isn't possible online, holding your hands up to look like you're touching the edge of your box can be a fun activity. Turn your palms out as if you're touching the hands of the people in the boxes next to you.

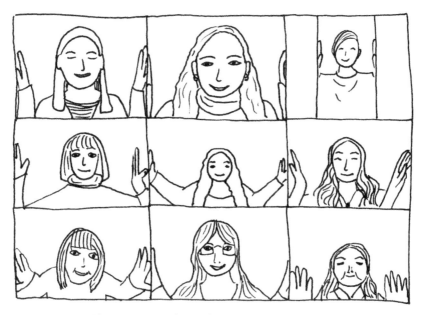

Figure 16.1 Hands together at end of online circle

Gemma Brady shared,

> In online circles, something I encourage people to do at the end of someone's share is to place their hand on their heart as acknowledgement. I will also state at the beginning of the circle that this gesture might feel strange. We don't have to look like we are listening online. The way of relating is different and that, I think, is the biggest challenge. I hold a lot of spaces online and find them to be just as potent. I don't find it as different as I thought it would.

Looking at your own face in an online circle can be disconcerting and is not necessary. It is possible to join an online Zoom circle and for others to be able to see you but remove yourself from 'self-view' (click on the three dots at the top right of your screen). We don't usually look at ourselves while sitting in circle time and there is no need for us to have to see ourselves online either!

In addition to using listening partnerships during the circle to create connection, you can also invite and facilitate people to use listening partnerships outside of the circle time. Make sure that they are clear on how the activity works, and we recommend that they agree on a specific time for talking (e.g. ten minutes each) and don't move into general conversation afterwards. If this happens, it takes more time and can lead to a regular partnership not being sustained.

Breaking up screen time

We want people to leave the circle feeling refreshed and so it's a good idea to build in time where participants are not looking at the screen. This can be during settling practices, which could be done a few times during the circle to provide a break with eyes closed or looking away from the screen. Any embodied practice can be done without the use of the screen if it is designed in a way where the person leading the practice does not need to be mirrored.

'Palming' is a great practice for this purpose. Invite people to rub their palms together to produce some warmth. Then place the palms gently over the eyes to let the warmth sink in. The hands can be still or some gentle pressure or circles can be added to relax the muscles around the eyes.

You can also explain that it will not be seen as rude if people want to look away from the screen and gaze at something further away to rest the eyes. Inviting people to practise 'orienting' is another useful way to soothe the nervous system. Ask people to look around the room, turning their head to look to the sides and even behind them. This can satisfy the primitive part of the brain that you are in a safe environment. Noticing what you can see, hear and physically feel brings you into the present moment and a feeling of being grounded back in your space.

> Online is different and it is the same. The framing is exactly the same. When you are facilitating online, you don't feel the energy in the same way. Do they need more time in breakout rooms? Do they need to be muted on the chat? Do they need a break? You still listen to what needs to happen.
>
> *Benedict Beaumont*

Screen time limits and breaks are important in an online gathering. We have found that two hours is manageable for most, especially if embodiment practices, movement, time away from screen and opportunities for breakout rooms with smaller groups are included. We have also found that limiting the number of participants to 12 in an online gathering will allow for all people to participate verbally. Larger gatherings would tend to limit verbal interaction and the chat (text box) for written interaction needs to be used more.

Checking in with people

With an online circle, it is much easier for someone to leave than it is in person. Checking in with someone is easier when you have more than one facilitator so that one can still hold the space and watch for the nuances in the talking, while the other can check in with one specific person. The chat facility on Zoom can be a useful way of communicating privately with someone who seems upset or disengaged. (Select the person's name in the drop-down box that you want to send a message to.) It is also useful if you are co-facilitating because you can chat to each other privately if timing is going astray or you need to adapt something in your circle schedule.

Part of the framing for the session would be to address what happens if you feel upset or triggered. Rather than leaving without explanation, set the expectation at the beginning that people share in the circle or privately that they are thinking of leaving. Check that people know how to use the private chat function and request that they give a brief explanation of why they are leaving so you are not worrying about them and know whether to follow up. (Perhaps they're leaving because it's an evening circle and their small child woke up and needs settling back to bed, in which case you wouldn't need to follow up.)

If someone does leave without explanation, we feel that the facilitator has a duty of care to the person and should get in touch through the contact details they have to check how the person is. This is why it is important to collect at least an email address when people sign up for a circle rather than posting a Zoom link publicly. It is easy to collect email addresses for people attending your meeting by using the registration function if you are opening a free circle. You can also cap numbers to ensure that there will be space for everyone to participate.

Depending on your group you can be specific about how people gain access to the Zoom link. You might have a registration process in place for people joining your organisation before they can attend a circle meeting. You may require people to speak to you or be involved with email correspondence before being invited to an online circle.

Hybrid online and in-person circles

Hybrid events can work well depending on what your circle includes. If movement is included, you will have to decide whether people online need to be able to see your movements clearly or can move from your description alone. A fisheye lens can be purchased that widens the view of the room you're in.

If you're using music, consider whether you need a licence to share it online. Some facilitators have the music playing on a separate device in their room. If you share it from the device you're also using for Zoom, you will need to select 'Share' and then tick 'Share sound' in the bottom left-hand corner.

You might need to consider a separate microphone that can be placed in the centre of the physical circle of people, or a microphone that is handed round like a talking stick, so that those online can clearly hear their voices.

To give you an example of how a hybrid event can work, Julia describes her quarterly yoga nidra event:

Yoga nidra (yoga sleep) is a deep relaxation practice. The event begins with a short settling practice and talking circle, giving people an opportunity to arrive, settle and speak.

A number of different people share a relaxation practice (the yoga nidra). These are recorded and the people online can hear the practice clearly as a laptop with a good microphone is used. After each practice, there is a talking circle with space to unpack the experience. Both people there in person and those online have the opportunity to speak and reflect.

When booking, it was clear to all participants that the event would take place both online and in person. To check that both online and in-person participants were happy with their experience, I ask for feedback. The recordings of the yoga nidras are available to everyone who booked.

We would recommend that you have some way of receiving and recording feedback too. Although it can feel daunting to ask how people found the experience, you will learn valuable insights that can improve your facilitation.

The next exercise gives you an opportunity to reflect on the points we've raised about facilitating online.

● EXERCISE: ONLINE CIRCLE TROUBLESHOOTING

Take a few minutes to read through the scenario and then consider the questions.

> You are invited to join an online circle. The theme has been clearly explained and the session begins with a short breathwork practice. You are each invited to share your experience and then you notice that the session is being recorded.

> For clarification, you ask about the recording: 'Who is the recording for? Who will it be shared with?' The facilitator is evasive and then you become aware that the circle is also being live-streamed without your permission on Facebook.

> By this time, your feelings of safety and security are being tested. You decide to not share and are not happy having your face shown publicly when you don't know who's watching.

> Others have turned off their videos. You don't know if that's because they don't want to be recorded either or because there are other people in the room with them.

> You decide to leave and are left feeling unsettled.

How could the facilitator have set up the online circle differently? How could they have responded differently when they realised someone wasn't feeling comfortable?

How would you have felt and what would you have done if you were the participant in this situation?

As a facilitator, what different skills have you noticed are needed to run online circles?

There is no limit to how big an online circle could be: its effectiveness will depend on how you create smaller spaces for people to connect with each other, as the next two stories show.

CIRCLE STORY: GLOBAL ONLINE CIRCLE

Gemma Brady shared with us a story of how circles can be effective even when they're online and large. She said:

> There is one [circle] in particular that stands out for quite different reasons. In 2020, I was asked by a large international company to run a circle for their end-of-year women's gathering.

> At the time, I was used to holding circles for between eight and ten people in person. I used to have a rule that I didn't hold any circles online. It was a really strong rule and then in December 2019 I had this funny feeling, maybe I should be experimenting online. The company said this circle was for 500 employees! My task was to sit with the question: 'Can I hold a circle-type space for people who will not have had experience of circle before?'

It was a big brief!

The event was for female employees from Europe, Africa and the Middle East. She found a way to hold that space by having a big group introduction and then doing work in smaller groups in breakout rooms.

The theme was around ancestral storytelling. She found online circles to be just as potent in different ways. She says:

> Online can be as connected and as powerful [as in person]. One of the challenges though about being online is that you are seeing everyone on the same screen and watching everyone's facial reactions in a way that you do not when you are sitting in a circle space in person.

> When you are sharing online you are seeing the flick of everyone's eye, what their resting face is, and from an emotional point of view it can be more challenging to share in that environment.

She suggests that if you find it off-putting to see your own face on screen, on Zoom you can use the function to remove your face from your own view. You can see everyone else in circle and they can see you, but you do not have to look at your own features and expressions.

Gemma says, 'The feedback from that circle and the feedback from that space was utterly mind-blowing... It was just astonishing to hold that many people.'

CIRCLE STORY: ADDRESSING A
NEED FOR CONNECTION

Lee Keylock of the organisation Narrative 4 shares the effect of the Covid pandemic on their circle and story exchange events:

> Most of our work had been in person. We were going into communities and people were face to face and then lockdown happened. We pivoted online very quickly and all of a sudden overnight we became very sought after because people had this emotional load that they wanted to release. They felt a need to be in community. The loneliness of the pandemic was huge. It still is. We still haven't recovered.

> I think we were providing a service to people where they could share stories and where the burden was lifted. People all over the world were showing up. Sometimes we capped them at 24 and we would have three facilitators in that space. It was an opportunity for people to unburden themselves. They got curious about each other and then they got imaginative and then they stayed in community with each other.

> It was more than likely that people who were partnered would stay in contact with each other because they had shared a special moment. Narrative 4 provided connection to people during the pandemic. People who felt isolated and lonely were given a valuable opportunity to make new connections and friendships.

With larger numbers, it is possible that more than one facilitator will be needed to create the container required for meaningful connection.

Being in a talking and listening circle generally involves being seen by others, so when running and participating in an online circle, the expectation to have your video on ensures that others know that you are fully participating and that nobody else is present. If people do not have their videos on, it can take away from another person's sense of safety and security.

As a facilitator, it is up to you to communicate the expectation around the online etiquette that you have decided is right for the people attending and the reason for meeting. An online circle can be an incredible resource for people who may not otherwise meet others with shared life experiences or interests.

In the next two chapters, we turn to the practical matters of marketing your circle, administration and logistics to make sure your event is a success.

CHAPTER 17

Spreading the Word and Filling Your Circle

You enjoyed hosting your first circle. Now you want to make this circle a regular gathering; you are thinking about how to spread the word about it, the language to use to explain what a talking circle is and is not, and how to make it sustainable emotionally as well as financially. You realise that facilitating a circle is not just about the time holding space during the gathering, but the supporting work around it too.

When you had the idea to start the talking circle, you might not have given much thought to how others would hear about it and imagined letting word spread organically. How much marketing you do might depend on whether you are running the circle as part of your work or as a hobby and whether you want to make a profit. In this chapter, we share tips on making your circle sustainable whatever your ambitions.

Marketing your circle

The container for the circle starts with how to tell your intended participants about the event. Sharing the guidelines and values to support kind communication in marketing material will be reassuring. You can also make it clear that speaking is not essential. If you have a heart-led need for circle time, you may be surprised by how easy it is to attract others who are also seeking what you are looking for.

Giving a brief outline of what happens within a circle is helpful too. For example:

We start with brief introductions, then have a settling practice where you can get used to the space. There is a topic to start off the talking with a poem or something else being read out and we see whether people connect to the theme and would like to share their experience. We close the circle on time, with a few words about how you found the circle.

A talking circle can have a long contemplation stage where people are weighing up the perceived pros and cons of attending. This is usually because they know communication will happen at a deeper level than normal and worry about being vulnerable. Speaking to these concerns supports people to attend. Having an option of a brief call to connect can make a massive difference in people feeling confident to book.

Creating a Facebook event or Eventbrite event can make it easily searchable in your local area. Otherwise, posting information about your circle where your intended audience gathers (in person or virtually) can be helpful. For example, if your group is for new parents, posting in a local parents Facebook group or putting a leaflet up at a weighing clinic or breastfeeding support group could help.

If you use Instagram, sharing a video of you explaining what happens in a circle can be helpful in breaking down barriers to people attending. If it's an online circle, you could run a taster, shorter circle to explain what happens and give potential participants a flavour of the event. If using an app like Zoom, remember to select Registration so that you have the email addresses to follow up with. You want to give people an opportunity to connect with you as the facilitator.

● EXERCISE: CREATING A CIRCLE FLYER/POST

Below is a template to spark ideas for your own circle. Consider whether different information would be needed.

Monthly Carers Meet-Up

The aim of the group is to have a space that
focuses on you and some time out.

There will be an opportunity to introduce yourself to the
others and find a relaxing activity to switch off for a while,
such as mindful colouring or decorating a keepsake box.

While we're sitting around, there is time to share about yourself: for
example, what would help you to relax, or what activities you did
before caring responsibilities. It's a chance to remember who you are

as well as a carer, in a respectful, non-judgemental and confidential environment. You don't need to share. Coming and listening is welcome.

Refreshments are provided.

Meets first Monday of every month. 10.00–11.30 a.m.

Contact [Name] at [email address] or [phone number]

Venue: [address]

FREE parking and £1 donation towards refreshments

If the circle is free or by donation, services or businesses are normally very happy for you to advertise by putting up a leaflet in their venue. If it is a paid event, don't be put off if they decline. Look for community boards in your local shopping area or supermarket.

If you are looking to start a circle, it is possible that you already know people who fit your 'who', people who are close and familiar to you like friends or family. If you start there, you can build your confidence and think through what works in a friendly environment. We have found when starting circles in our local area, inviting friends and neighbours first has worked well and word of mouth has spread from there.

Much is made of creating marketing materials, but if you are looking to run something local for your community, word of mouth can go a long way. This is especially true if you are creating a circle for a demographic that you are part of.

For a very specific group of people or interest, you may need a presence on the internet to be able to find those who are spread out geographically. When Julia recently lost cousins in a terrorist attack, she looked for an organisation that might be able to support her in her grief. Because of the traumatic circumstances of the deaths, she looked very specifically for a circle where the trauma of the experience would be understood by those who had experienced it.

If you already offer other classes or services like yoga, meditation, reflex-ology or tai chi, don't be shy about telling people about this new offering. In these cases, people may be willing to try something that is normally out of their comfort zone because of the 'know, like and trust' factor that they have with you. Both Julia and Tessa include circle time in their workshops, and there is considerable crossover in their yoga and circle-holding audiences.

Template: Online circle email invitation
Read through this example, and if you're a movement teacher or somebody else with an existing client base, think how you could adapt the email for your own purposes.

Hi [Name]

Thank you for attending my classes. I'm so happy that you enjoy them.
I wanted to let you know about a new event I'm organising that you might be interested in.
For the last couple of years, I have been attending a NAME OF CIRCLE [that you have been attending] and it has become the highlight of my month. It's such a special space that I can relax into and just be me. I love the respectful listening that happens as people are sharing.
On [date], I will be hosting the first NAME OF CIRCLE. It will run for two hours from [time]. We will start with some easy introductions, then have a short breathing practice to settle. Then I'll introduce the topic, which will be about connecting with what lights up your heart.
At the end, we'll close with a simple check-in and have time for socialising.
If you're thinking, 'I would love that. Sign me up!' book here [link].
Or if you're curious, but a little unsure, hit reply and let's arrange a time to talk after class or a ten-minute phone call.
I hope you'll get as much as I do out of circle time.

[Your name]

Bookings and joining information

Depending on the size of your business or if this is a hobby, there are different options for taking bookings. You might simply keep a list of who has signed up via emails or said they will attend via social media platforms. It's important to take at least their name and email address so that you have a way of contacting them if the event is cancelled or they don't show up, and to tell them about the next event. Consent is required for any taking of email addresses in the UK (Data Protection Act 2018), so it is important to ask their permission, and you may also be required to pay a fee to the Data Protection Commission to store the names (see ico.org.uk/fee-self-assessment).

If you don't use an email platform, then having a password-protected spreadsheet of contact details would be ideal.

If you are not charging for your circle, then it can be helpful for people to know if you limit numbers so that they are aware that if they book and then do not attend, they are potentially taking a place away from someone else. For example, 'Please note: If you book a place and for some reason your circumstances change and you are unable to join the circle, please let the office know as soon as possible so that your place can be offered to someone else.'

If you run a number of events, using a booking system saves time. Platforms like Eventbrite, Ticket Tailor, website booking plugins and specialist systems like Reservie for yoga teachers cost money (a percentage of the ticket price or a monthly fee), but make keeping track of attendees and sending out confirmation emails much easier for a growing business.

In the UK, there are specific compliance issues as soon as you start taking paid bookings. Details about data compliance and other issues when collecting information for payment can be found at the Information Commission Office (https://ico.org.uk). Many of the booking and email management platforms have GDPR (General Data Protection Regulation) built into their systems to make sure that you comply with the Data Protection Act.

Once someone has booked, we recommend sending a confirmation email with joining instructions (see an example email below). Think about all the information that someone will need:

- date, start and finish times

- clear directions to the venue, including instructions on parking and public transport (also lift-sharing opportunities)

- what to bring (e.g. a mug, food to share, cushions, blanket, pen and paper if you're planning journalling, layers of clothing if you're sitting outside, objects for the centrepiece, crafts)

- cancellation policy in case of illness or bad weather (if it's an outside circle)

- reminder of the guidelines and values of the circle

- contact information for the facilitator in case they're running late

- if online, the link to join the virtual meeting.

Template: Confirmation email for circle event

Dear [Name]

I am looking forward to welcoming you to:

NAME OF CIRCLE

DATE and TIME OF CIRCLE

This is a place for you to be seen, held and heard.

The purpose of the circle is to: ....

By attending, you will [list benefits connected to the aim of the circle]

Preparing for the circle

We won't be doing any movement in this circle, so please wear whatever you're most comfortable in.

You might like to bring:

- a blanket for getting cosy

- a pen and paper

- Something to share (your favourite tea, biscuits) – OPTIONAL

Warmly

[YOUR NAME]

Terms & Conditions [If applicable. Recommended if there is a fee to attend.]

[e.g. We do not provide refunds or exchanges for future events due to internet issues, late arrival, issues with regard to finding emails or time zone issues. Cancellations within 7 days of the event are non-refundable.]

If the event has a long lead time, sending a reminder or the joining instructions in the week before the circle will support people to attend. If there are spaces still available, you can also include an invitation to bring a friend who is interested.

If you're someone who actively dislikes marketing, try to reframe it as spreading the word about the valuable service that you are offering. Go back and look at Chapters 3 and 4 – the exercises in these chapters will help you create marketing that will feel authentic. You could approach places that already have established networks such as community centres and yoga studios (if your circle is relevant to these venues) and ask them if they will tell people on their mailing lists. Beware, though, that this can leave you in a precarious situation as the people attending are primarily clients or users of the venue and you are unlikely to have direct access to their email addresses. Communicating directly with the community about what you're passionate about is always going to have the best impact.

In the next chapter, we will look at the practicalities of running free, by donation and paid-for circles. We will look at reasons why you might wish to choose each model and how to introduce and structure payment.

CHAPTER 18

Paid and Unpaid Circles and Preventing Burnout

You know who your circle is for and what the aim of the talking is. Now you need to make the decision about whether your circle is free to attend or attendance by donation, or whether a charge is needed to cover your costs and time. There is your energy to consider and how this fits in with other work and the rest of your life.

Paid and unpaid circles

Whether you wish to charge for your circle depends on your own needs, wants and costs. Should it be a set cost, a sliding scale, by donation or free to attend? The answer is 'It depends!' It depends on whether the people you intend to come to your circle can afford to pay for such an event. Are you running this as a business (and there's nothing wrong with that) or as a hobby? If you are embarking on this enterprise yourself, you may wish to ask yourself whether charging or asking for donations will make the circle more sustainable in the long term.

Another reason for charging is that making a financial commitment can affect attendance positively. Abbey shared, 'When I created my first circle I had the clarity that I needed to charge. When I experimented with deviating from this, I found that the numbers dwindled due to lack of commitment.'

Some believe that when people pay for something, they tend to value it more. In some cases that may be true. We have both attended paid-for and free circles and valued them equally. When Julia attended free SAMM meetings she highly valued the circle support provided. The circles are run by volunteers, all of whom have been trained by the organisation and have experience of attending their circles and retreats. It was clear from their words that the women attending the free Gather the Women circle also valued the existence of the group. Alcoholic Anonymous (AA) meetings are free and provide a lifeline to the recovery community. All the above organisations are supported via a strong infrastructure in order to be sustainable emotionally and financially.

We will first look at deciding whether your circle is to be paid for by the participants attending, by donation or free to attend. Then, later in the chapter, we will explore other options for financing talking and listening circles.

● EXERCISE: ALIGNING INTENTIONS AND FINANCIAL SUPPORT

Take a moment to read through the questions and reflect on your responses. There is no morally superior choice to be made here: it is about deciding what will make your circle sustainable.

Free to attend

- Are there venue, refreshment or craft materials costs that you will incur? Do you have childcare costs of your own to cover?

- If you're running the circle in your home, are there extra energy costs that you need to consider? Can you afford the extra amount? Is there someone else at home that might feel differently?

- Could you move around participants' homes to share energy costs?

- Can you ask people to take turns bringing refreshments?

- Is your income sufficient from other work to cover your time facilitating the circle? (Remember not just the time holding the circle, but also preparing and marketing it.)

By donation

- What costs do you need to be covered by the donations received? The outlay for basic costs of venue, refreshments and craft materials, or also for your time and expertise?

- Will you suggest an amount of donation that supports you to run this circle? Can you share some of the costs involved in a confirmation email to help people make their decision?

- How will you collect the donation to give people anonymity? If the circle is online, can you set up a donation option using a payment system?

- Could you receive donations other than monetary ones? These could be for products or services, such as a massage for every three or four circles attended.

Paid for

- How much would cover the basic costs such as venue, refreshments and booking fees?

- How much extra would take account of the time preparing and running the circle, that makes you feel good about the work?

- Can you offer a sliding scale for people to choose the amount they can afford?

- Would a concessionary rate work well, or a helper position that is a lower cost or free?

- Do you feel that people will have higher expectations of a paid circle? Is that affecting your reflections about whether to charge or not?

- If you have a co-facilitator, will you share equally the profits from the circle or do you have different roles with varying amounts of workload?

- Have you discussed and recorded your decisions clearly?

- Are there already offerings for this demographic in the area? Does your pricing reflect what is commonly paid for similar offerings?

Now return to your intentions for the circle in Chapter 3. Is your intention to run a regular circle? Although it may seem strange to consider the long term when you've not even run your first circle, how would you feel in one year about running a monthly circle and all the work involved if it was free or by donation? Would the satisfaction be enough?

You can run a first circle for free or by donation as a trial run. Use it as an opportunity to build your confidence and gain feedback. Ask for testimonials if people enjoyed it and to gauge whether the amount of donations (if requested) is sufficient. Showing people the value of the circle may build your ability to request payment.

To make a circle sustainable, it may be necessary to charge to attend. Burnout is a real consideration when running circles because they can involve a big amount of work for little return or even a loss if you haven't thought through the financial implications.

You might decide to run an inclusive business where nobody is turned away for economic reasons or you may choose to offer a sliding scale of costs so that discounts are afforded to people from specific demographics. In our experience, it is rare that people abuse sliding scales or concessionary rates. Although there may be people who abuse the system, it is far more likely that you will be opening up your circle to people who might otherwise be unable to afford it.

> There are monthly subscriptions and it is done by direct debit but I am sensitive to who is worrying about money. The idea is absolute equality of opportunity. I try to get to know the parents sufficiently so I know if [there's a financial issue]... I have a discretionary fund for extras like trips or equipment like wellies so nobody realises we've helped out.
>
> *George, youth leader*

It is okay to charge for the time and effort you take to create a circle.

The next exercise goes into greater detail about the potential costs involved in facilitating a circle, including those that may be shared with other activities such as professional insurance and website fees. To reflect the true cost of holding a circle, all of these should be considered.

● EXERCISE: WHAT SHOULD I CHARGE?

This is a common question in our training courses. Rather than looking around to see what others charge, first work through which of these potential costs will apply to your circle to see what outlay you have before you add the value of your time and experience.

Some of the costs will be proportional: that is, if you include website fees in your calculations, you might only include a small amount if you use your website for other activities. If you do not know the exact amount, use an estimation.

Cost

- Venue (include time for set-up and tidying away)
- Your own transport (petrol, parking, bus ticket)

- Your childcare costs or if offering to participants

- Refreshments

- Energy costs (e.g. if facilitating at home)

- Booking fees (if using booking platform)

- Website and hosting costs (a proportion of)

- Marketing costs (e.g. printing leaflets)

- Zoom fees (free version only gives you 45 minutes)

- Music licence fee (if relevant)

- Disclosure and Barring Service (DBS) check fee (if working with children or vulnerable adults)

- Insurance cost (where relevant)

- Professional membership (e.g. for yoga teachers, if also teaching yoga as part of event)

- Training costs

- Craft materials

- Materials for a centrepiece or other decoration

- Printed materials if using colouring or handouts

- Relevant books

- Setting-up costs (e.g. mugs, cushions, blankets)

- Other:

TOTAL: . . . .

The total above will give you an idea of your outlay and how much you need to charge to avoid running your circle at a loss. Some of these costs, like training, will be spread over a number of circles if you plan to run them regularly.

Now consider the value of your time and experience. If you find this difficult, ask someone who has attended circles or another circle holder to support your thinking around this.

How do you feel about running the circle for free, for a donation or charging at the end of this exercise?

In deciding whether to charge or not, and how much, it's important to reflect on what amount will help you to feel positive about facilitating the talking circle over time. In deciding the value of the circle, you support others to understand its value too. A well-facilitated talking circle can look like an easy activity to run, but from reading this book you know how much work happens behind the scenes.

CIRCLE STORY: TESSA'S EXPERIENCE OF CHARGING

At the time of writing, Tessa has been running her women's circle for ten years: starting in a venue where she taught yoga classes, switching to her living room when the former didn't feel cosy enough, moving to a yurt when the circle became bigger, then online during the pandemic and back to her living room. At first, it was called a Red Tent and so she honoured the principle of attendance by donation. Over a two-year period of doing this, it was clear that what people gave varied considerably. This would sometimes mean that the cost of the venue (yoga space/yurt) wouldn't be covered.

Tessa has observed that there is a pattern where those who are themselves self-employed tend to give more when donating than those who are employed and have a regular salary. Perhaps this is because they know the supporting work that goes into running your business. One approach could be to give a guide cost even if your preference is for people to donate so that they know the value of a place at the event.

When Tessa switched to a set cost (but with concessions available), she found that the group became more stable. Asking people to pay for their place on booking meant that they still attend when there is adverse weather or they have had a stressful day. Once they arrive, people are glad they made the effort!

If there is a cancellation, she uses her discretion about whether to move the booking over to the next circle or whether someone has lost their fee. (The terms and conditions state that the fee is non-refundable, but sometimes she offers to transfer the booking when it is due to difficult circumstances.) When you have a bigger circle with a waiting list, if someone doesn't give you enough time to invite someone in their place, others have missed out.

One of the main factors that means the circle has run continuously for ten years is that Tessa started charging for it so that all her costs are covered, including her time facilitating and administering the event. She says:

> I feel that what I do is so valued by the people who attend. There have been people who attended regularly who were having a hard time financially and so they came for free for some months. There is flexibility when you charge and so I have never felt resentful about running it or that I'm excluding people.

In addition to the women's in-person circle and circle holders' online gatherings, she runs more informal, free talking gatherings that are a springboard to find out about other services that she offers. She also uses a very basic form of circle time in her yoga classes to provide a simple check-in at the beginning of class and facilitate connection. She shares, 'Talking and listening circles are such a beautiful way of creating community. I can't imagine life without them now!'

You may be planning to run your talking and listening circle under the umbrella of an organisation, in which case they might have stipulations around charging. For example, the Red Tent Directory (https://redtent-directory.com) stipulate that Red Tents should be free or by donation: '[Red Tents are] gatherings which are either free or donation-based to cover room hire or tea with the amount ideally left to the discretion of the donor.' Likewise, when the Positive Birth Movement groups were running, the founder stipulated that they should be free to attend and not involve pushing of facilitators' services like pregnancy yoga, doula hire or hypnobirthing courses.

Facilitating a free circle can be a conscious decision to create a springboard to other events. Both Tessa and Julia run a mix of paid-for and free circles. The free circles work well as an introduction to circle holding practices and the yoga trainings they provide. For Julia, they give space for participants to discover more about her Yoga Teachers Forum organisation: to talk about and experience embodiment practices that connect them to their role as yoga teachers and may wish to develop. For Tessa, she offers Healthy Mum Meet Ups that act as a springboard to local mum and baby yoga classes, learning hypopressive exercises and birth trauma yoga sessions. Over time, they have found the right balance of unpaid offerings and paid work.

If you are unsure about running your circles alone, joining an organisation that provides training and support could be an excellent option. Gather the Women (www.gatherthewomen.org) is a non-profit organisation that is run by volunteers. Donations can be made through the website to support their work but no payment is directly taken for attending a circle.

Many charities use circle work to support their communities. Often people who have experienced a specific trauma are trained to support others who have experienced something similar. In Support after Murder and Manslaughter (SAMM) events, the online circles are held by volunteers who receive specific training and gift their time. During our research we have found many free circles.

If you are a movement teacher working for a yoga studio, adult education college or other organisation, you could collaborate with others to create a circle to build community. This is invaluable for creating a loyal group who attend not only for enjoyment of the activity but also for the friendships that build. When you work in collaboration with others, the workload will be shared.

CIRCLE STORY: THE CREATION OF THE YOGA TEACHERS FORUM

Julia began running a yoga teachers circle at her studio because as a self-employed woman she felt the need to connect with other teachers in her local community. This began with another teacher she knew, arranging a time for them to go round to someone's house, share a practice and chat informally. There was no structure to the gathering, it happened if and when teachers could gather, and the purpose of each gathering, other than to bring them together, was unfocused. Soon the meetings fizzled out.

A friend ran a large yoga studio near to her. This was the perfect location for them to come together as she had a bespoke space that would work for a group who would like to practise as well as talk. They would often gather, just the two of them, but there never seemed to be a right time and place for the teachers' circle.

She shares:

I decided it was time to create a circle myself. I solved the problem of the unstructured nature of the circle by planning to run the circle monthly on a Wednesday afternoon at my small studio space. To create a purpose for the circle, I decided to invite a yoga teacher with a different area of discipline each month to share their practice.

Timewise I chose to keep the session to two hours. At the time I was not using regular circle skills in the group. While it fulfilled its function to bring yoga teachers together, and the educational content ensured that teachers came, we had little time to really get to know each other as the session was filled with teaching, practice and questions.

I originally saw the monthly sessions as valuable to me as well as others so chose not to charge for them. Later, I decided that in order for people to commit there needed to be a level of financial commitment, so I asked for a voluntary donation of £5, rising to £10 over time, with all money going to charity. By the time I had been running the circle for two years it had begun to serve its purpose of connecting me to a number of local yoga teachers, a number of whom became trusted friends and colleagues. I found that the connections that I made ensured it was easy for me to find cover for my classes when I needed it and I no longer felt lonely.

I created a WhatsApp group of London teachers and felt that a sense of community was building. However, over time I began to resent the huge amount of work I did monthly to ensure the gatherings took place. Fellow yoga teachers began to encourage me to charge for the monthly sessions.

I found it really difficult to move from a place of charity donation-based offering to charging for the huge amount of time, effort and energy it took to maintain the meetings. I also held sole responsibility for the meetings and had no fellow teacher to support me as I held this space for the community.

Over time I realised that running a monthly, in-person teachers' circle with an education component was extremely time-consuming. There was considerable work that needed to be done to bring in a different teacher each month to share teaching and to encourage teachers to come along each month. While it felt good to be donating to local charity, I began to feel a little burnt out by the work.

I began to run paid-for events for teachers, alongside the teachers circle, and then the pandemic came along and everything went online.

This was the seed of the Yoga Teachers Forum. There was a significant benefit to the local teaching community of running the teachers 'circles' and I still run them on more of an ad hoc basis and when

I run them as free events they are online so there is a significantly lighter workload.

Julia's story about the creation of the Yoga Teachers Forum shows how founding a circle can be the initiation of something much bigger. The Celebration Day for Girls circles have become an international phenomenon, through careful thought about quality training and a percentage of the profit for the first few years feeding back into the organisation. You may be ambitious with your intentions for your circle and the needs you've identified. In the next story we hear an example about how to scale up.

CIRCLE STORY: CREATING AN INTERNATIONAL ORGANISATION

Narrative 4 is an organisation that started in the United States and aims to build inclusivity and connectedness through their circle time and story exchanges, whether in classrooms or boardrooms. Lee Keylock explains:

> It started with angel investors who believed in what we were doing. Amazon is a big funder of ours. We work with some corporate organisations. We want all of our money to go into programmes. We are also a very neutral organisation in the sense that we don't take political positions on things. We are not going to let anyone get hurt in the room. We are not going to take a position on people's stories. Their truth is their truth, however that is relayed, and we tie that to our fundraising messaging too.
>
> At the beginning it was mostly volunteer. If we go into a school we train teachers [to facilitate story exchanges]. If we do story exchanges for an organisation we pay facilitators. We have lead trainers. We have master practitioners.
>
> One of the big things for me is you cannot just run into any neighbourhood and say, 'Tell your story,' and then run away. For me, part of the infrastructure meant we have to do this in schools because there are many touchpoints you can have with children over years. That is how you build community and that is where change happens. Seventy per cent of our work is in schools because there is an infrastructure there.
>
> If you want to scale with integrity and intention then you have to have an infrastructure.

This story shows that when a circle concept becomes bigger, structure in terms of training and consistent communication is important. Where an existing infrastructure can be used, like schools, hospitals or prisons, then there is an opportunity to have a big impact more quickly.

These examples show that massive impact is possible with circle spaces. Whether it's one circle in your living room or a global network of circles, caring for yourself as a facilitator is crucial. Burnout is real and can happen due to both financial and emotional burden. We love running circles and know that in order to sustain this work we need to care for ourselves, both financially and emotionally.

Alternative models

You may choose to facilitate with others to share the workload and costs involved. A totally collaborative model could see you taking turns to facilitate in your own home without any money changing hands. There are many benefits of collaborating in this way: for example, you bring more inspiration and skills into the circle; you have frequent opportunities to be a participant as well as a facilitator; there is a real equalisation of power; and if you are ill, the circle can go ahead.

Andrew shares:

> It was egalitarian. Everyone had their own roles. Someone I have known since I was four years old and I am still friends with today, he always wanted to light the fire. He would build us a good old fire. Other people would be sorting out things to sit on. You could bet who would do each thing.

Issues to consider of shared collaboration are: the possibility of losing direction without a designated leader (e.g. who is responsible for setting dates and communicating them?); not everyone having a suitable home space to facilitate (could they do an outdoor circle in the summer months?); differing levels of facilitation skill or experience (could they buddy up with someone who is more confident?); the lack of charging leading to informality and lack of circle boundaries. This is not a finite list of benefits or challenges, so we invite you to reflect on others that may be relevant for the demographic or specific focus for your planned circle.

In practice, we've found that it can take a little time to settle into a cohesive group where everyone is willing to step up to facilitate in this way. It may be that one person has to take on an organising role to begin with – for example, setting up a WhatsApp group to communicate and taking the initiative to host the first event.

A different model is volunteering for a charity or other organisation that uses circle spaces. In some cases, such as SAMM, the circles are run by volunteers in rotation with others so that you are sharing the facilitation. The organisations take responsibility for marketing the circle and often facilitators are trained free of charge. We have learned many lessons from these circle facilitators during our research.

Setting up a charity is a huge undertaking, the description of which is outside the remit of this book. If you are looking to run circles based on this model, we highly recommend you look at the contacts and resources we share at the back of this book and find out more about how to set up a charity and create circles in this way. Read the circle story ' Becoming mums and the mothers' quilt' in Chapter 13 which is moving from a not-for-profit organisation to a charity at the time of writing.

Another way to be paid for running circles without taking payment from the attendees themselves is to apply for funding from your local council or a charity, or for grants like the National Lottery. The time taken to research what funding is available and to apply needs to be factored in, but this can be done very successfully. This could be appropriate for circles for any minority groups or with limited resources. Funding can guarantee you a wage for the circle you are holding without the onus being on the demographic you serve to pay you directly. Many religious organisations work in this way, providing services to their community indirectly paid for by people who share the faith.

If you already work within an organisation and wish to set up a circle within it, you may want to look at what burden that puts on you. Reflect on whether it is reasonable for you to facilitate a circle as part of your salaried workload. Perhaps the organisation will see the value in paying for you to have further training in circle facilitation to enhance your skill set. If you are looking to introduce circle time in a business environment, we recommend the book *The Circle Way* by Christina Baldwin and Ann Linnea (2010).

Asking for feedback

Whatever model you have decided on, asking for feedback is advisable. You will learn so much from what participants share. Once you have begun running your circles, it is helpful for you to gather feedback: it could be anonymous post-it notes at the end of the event, an email after the circle or sending a follow-up message on the platform from which people have been communicating with you.

Feedback can also be a wonderful way of obtaining testimonials to share in your future marketing. Make sure that you ask permission before sharing and check whether someone is happy to put their name or initials to the words or prefers it to be anonymous.

As we come to the end of this chapter, we hope that you have found it useful to consider in detail the workload and costs that may be involved in circle facilitation. In our circle-holding discussions we have heard from facilitators who began to feel resentful after running free circles for years. This is often the case when someone is not supported by a larger organisation and is finding that running the circle is coming at a greater cost to them both financially and emotionally than they anticipated or are able to hold. In order to run circles ourselves, we find that it is essential to earn sufficiently to be in a position to support ourselves through supervision, training and self-care to prevent burnout.

Our hope is that you realise the incredible service that you offer when you are a circle holder and that being paid for facilitation, whether it comes directly from the attendees or not, is valid and acceptable.

In the next chapter, we look at the practical logistics of running a talking and listening circle, such as finding an appropriate venue.

CHAPTER 19

Venue, Lighting and Other Practical Considerations

You know who the circle is for and how you want it to feel. Now you need to find a venue that contributes physically to creating a container for people to share. You want somewhere not too big and not too small, just like Goldilocks! Sometimes we can find the perfect space and other times we need to work with what we can find by changing the lighting and decoration.

In this chapter, we will share the different aspects of venues to consider, the impact of lighting and other practical considerations when planning a talking and listening circle. We have also included a checklist for what to prepare.

Venue considerations

Between us, we have run in-person circles in the lounge at home, a yoga studio, community halls, classrooms, a yurt, on retreat, outside next to willow trees and at festivals in a tepee. Talking circles can be run anywhere, but it's worth reflecting on how the environment will affect how comfortable physically and mentally people will be to share.

In general, an easily accessible venue where people will be comfortable is essential: temperature-wise, seating arrangements, access to toilets, the possibility to make tea, transport links, accessibility and parking. It also needs to be financially viable, so sometimes we need to compromise: a stylish venue may make the cost too expensive for participants (for a paid event).

For talking circles, being able to create a cosy, intimate space supports sharing. Tessa first tried running her women's circle in a venue where she likes teaching yoga, but it felt too big a space for a talking circle, even with blankets draped over seating and lower lighting.

Physical comfort is important. For example, if someone is cold and finds sitting on the floor awkward, then they are more likely to be focused on their physical needs than wanting to join the flow of talking. Psychological comfort is also essential. For example, if someone is joining a circle at a festival where people keep coming in and out, they may feel that they cannot share fully because they feel vulnerable.

Sometimes a venue is chosen for convenience, such as in a classroom during the lunch hour, but other times it might be chosen because it provides that feeling of having moved into a different kind of space from everyday life. Circles in yurts can be special for this reason, even more so if they are out in nature. There is a balance to be struck. Is your circle inclusive while being in an unusual place or natural setting? Considering accessibility, public transport, the potential for lift shares or whether someone with mobility challenges could attend is important.

Our advice would be to visit the venue at the time you want to host your circle. If it's a community space, there may be sound coming from other activities like loud music from a Zumba class, or perhaps the car park is already full of other visitors. Look at whether there are easy local transport links and any extra costs to participants for parking. These are all details you will need to share with them before booking.

If it's a regular circle that you intend to hold, check whether you will have keys, if you need to have someone to let you in or if you need to pick up keys from a key safe or a key holders' address each time. The latter can add considerable time to running the event.

Another consideration is whether the space is usually filled with furniture. If you need to clear the space or rearrange the furniture each time, this will add additional time. This is often the case in school or village halls, where although chairs and tables may be around the outside of the space, they can make it feel functional rather than cosy. Moving them closer together and perhaps bringing along cushions to make the chairs more comfortable could improve the setting.

You might have a pop-up space in the form of a bell tent, gazebo or yurt. For example, Cecilia Allon describes how 'The first time I held circle, I offered a red tent at a festival. I got myself a red bell tent, lots of books about menstruality, colouring books... I curated the space.' Tessa created a mini Red Tent space with a gazebo at her daughter's primary school space with blankets and cushions on the floor. It was a popular space to hang out.

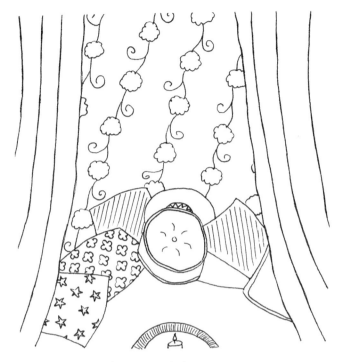

Figure 19.1 Circle time in a tent

Financial considerations are important too. Speak to the person respon-sible for the space and find out whether you will also need to pay for set-up and take-down time. Also check whether a deposit is required to hire the space or to be a key holder. The financial risk of running a circle in your living room is very different to hiring a venue.

The next exercise takes you through different considerations when choosing a venue. Remember that it does not have to be a perfect space, but 'good enough'.

EXERCISE: VENUE CHECKLIST

Go through the points and see whether they are relevant to your circle.

- Location (is it easily attractive, accessible?)

- Cost (business or community prices?)

- Deposit required (how long to get this back?)

- Access to building (is it obvious, safe, keyholder?)

- Accessibility for people with mobility issues
- Suitable seating for people with mobility issues
- Alarm to deactivate
- Sole or multiple use of venue
- Parking (off-street, on street, free or not?)
- Seating (enough for everyone, comfortable?)
- Lighting (can it be turned down for circle?)
- Temperature (can you control this in the venue?)
- Toilets (compost toilets okay for your attendees?)
- Kitchen or other way to make hot drinks
- Outside space
- Allowed to have candles
- Access to cleaning equipment (e.g. brush/vacuum cleaner)
- Professional insurance required (e.g. if yoga teacher)
- Other insurance required
- Certificate of training required (if relevant)

You might not be able to find the perfect venue and this shouldn't stop you from holding the circle. If the only venue you can find has uncomfortable plastic chairs, it's perfectly acceptable to ask people to bring cushions to make them more comfortable or to supply yoga mats and sit on those with cushions if your attendees have the mobility for this. Lighting is an important consideration and is covered in the section ' Lighting your circle space' below.

Hosting a circle in your home

I held [the circle] in my living room and I lived at the bottom floor of a former local authority building, so it wasn't very fancy. I had this tiny living room painted black that I made beautiful with candles...what happened in practice is that it felt like a real reclamation of my home space for something beautiful.

Gemma Brady

Holding a circle in your home can make for a cosy space. There can be benefits and drawbacks to facilitating in your own living space. Some of the benefits are that you will probably have more control over the space than other places and can decorate it however you wish, there isn't a hire fee and there is no travel time or cost for you. For the participants, it can feel special to be invited into someone's home, whereas a hire venue can feel impersonal.

One of the disadvantages is that there may be other people affected by your use of the space, such as family or housemates within your home and neighbours outside of it. Checking whether members of the household are willing to stay out of the way and quiet during the circle will be important for creating the container for the event. There are also bureaucratic considerations like whether the terms of your home insurance will be affected.

Having the circle in your space might make it feel special, as Gemma found, or over time it might come to feel like the boundary between work and personal life is blurred. There is no one right answer to these questions and it might change over time.

Lighting your circle space

A big impact on the atmosphere for your circle can be created through good lighting. Soft or natural lighting helps create an intimate space, whereas strip lighting makes it harder for the hormone of connection, oxytocin, to flow and can make people feel exposed.

If you are holding a circle when it is dark, it is worth the time to visit a venue at that time ahead of the gathering to check the effect that the lighting has. You might be able to take table lamps to create a softer atmosphere or add fairy lights or LED candles (without making it too dark that faces can't be clearly seen) to create a magical atmosphere.

Tessa has learnt from experience to check the lighting beforehand. A mum had chosen a nursery space for her mother blessing when pregnant with her fourth child. There was a fabulous big sofa and great seating, but no way to soften the lighting: it was either pitch black or fluorescent strip lighting. Tessa says:

I knew the venue from taking my own children there, but I'd only ever been there during daylight hours. It's a lovely light space with high ceilings. I had never noticed that only strip lighting was available and it was too harsh.

If she'd visited the venue in the evening ahead of the event, she would have known to take some table lamps.

Using only candles and firelight could be magical after people have had the chance to connect and create a feeling of safety within their nervous systems. However, it may feel unsafe to others because it tends to be shifting and low-level light. If you advertise your circle as 'candlelit', then an expectation will be set for low lighting. Considering who is attending your circle is important and you can check in with people after they arrive too.

In the same way, it can be magical to sit around a fire outside for most people. Having only the light from the fire at night can bring a feeling of intimacy and being part of something ancient. Matt Walker shares, 'Those sort of campfire discussions were brilliant...it was quite therapeutic. People joined in and said things that they never in a million years would have spilled the beans about in daylight.'

When deciding whether or not to hold a circle in an outdoor setting, once again advance warning is recommended. In the early evening in the UK, for example, those who experience hay fever can be particularly affected and mosquitos are also more likely to be around. Advance warning gives people the opportunity to choose whether the set-up is attractive to them and to wear suitable clothing.

Israh Goodall described:

Often we sit around a fire. A hearth is a place we can all return to. We can all remember this is why we are here. Symbolically, we can share a piece of wood in the fire. Shared intention brings us together.

For other people, it may be the first time they've had this experience and the elemental nature of fire could feel frightening. As circle holders, we may sometimes want to give people a new experience and we can support people's nervous systems by sharing in advance what the set-up will be. Of course, for some events you may wish to have surprises in store, but it's important to indicate if you are planning to put people out of their comfort zone. Some will be excited by this and others will not.

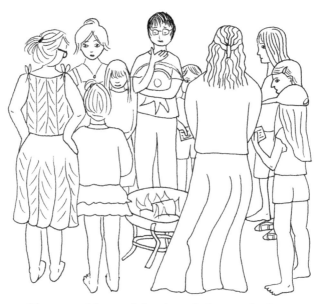

Figure 19.2 Mum and daughter circle around a fire

Decorating the circle space

In Chapter 5, we shared ideas about how to set up your space to create the right atmosphere for your gathering. Depending on the venue you are using, you might need to work hard to change the feeling of the space. Some venues have stipulations about not sticking things on the wall and not being able to use electrical items like lights that haven't been tested for safety.

Kate Forde, a dedicated circle holder, takes one hour to set up the space with mats, bolsters, blankets and cushions that she provides herself and then another hour to pack up afterwards. She says, 'It takes ages, but it's what people come for. It's what makes my events different from other people's. I love creating a nurturing space so it's worth the extra time.'

You also need a big car to transport all of these props. The time taken to set up and pack up should be included in how you cost the event and will be factored into the hiring cost for most venues.

You may also need to clean the space before you can set up. For example, if you're using a school or community hall, brushing or vacuuming the floor might be necessary before you can set out your circle. Check that you have access to the right equipment, and if it happens on a regular basis, talk to the venue administrator.

Even if your circle is online, you can still think about the space that you are sitting in. Consider what the background looks like, tidying it and perhaps putting something behind you that is relevant. You can also use the background filter on Zoom to obscure what's behind you. Perhaps you want to light a candle or make the space feel special to you. You can invite the circle attendees to do the same and perhaps share in the circle how they set up for the gathering, or show their lit candle, flowers or other collected items.

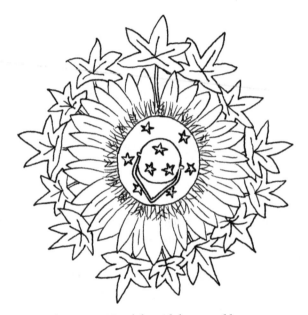

Figure 19.3 Mandala with lamp and leaves

Below is a checklist of items you might need. This is a long list and you may need very few of them. If you continue to run regular circles, you may choose to add more resources.

EXERCISE: CHECKLIST OF ITEMS FOR IN-PERSON CIRCLE

See which of these are relevant to you. For a regular circle, you could create your own checklist of frequently needed items to speed up the preparation.

Administration/resources

- List of people's names and contact numbers

- Emergency contact number for venue
- List of services to signpost to
- Reading/poem
- Relevant books
- Schedule with timings

Decoration/seating

- Lighting: table lamps, fairy lights, LED candles
- Items for centrepiece (e.g. material and candle)
- Matches/lighter
- Throws/shawls for walls or sofas
- Cushions/bolsters/meditation chairs/blanket

Refreshments

- Mugs/glasses
- Teas, milk, sugar, squash
- Snacks (any allergies?)
- Tissues

Activities

- Talking stick or other object
- Device to play music
- Craft materials
- Scissors/glue
- Paper and pens (if journalling – some people will always forget theirs)
- Tealights for people to light their own candle
- Coloured card in small shapes – write people's closing word and place around centrepiece
- Instrument to make sound with (e.g. hand chimes, singing bowl)

Things to remind people to bring

- Eyeglasses (e.g. if sewing, remind people to bring their glasses)
- Comfortable clothing
- Cushions/blanket
- Food to share
- Mug or water bottle
- Torch (if circle is in nature)

EXERCISE: CHECKLIST OF ITEMS FOR ONLINE CIRCLE

Here is a list of suggested items for you to bring and also to invite your participants to have ready.

Administration/resources

- List of people's names and contact numbers
- List of services to signpost to
- Reading/poem
- Relevant books
- Schedule with timings

Decoration/seating

- Lighting so that people can see your face clearly
- Tidy background or use filter
- Candle/flowers to make it special for you

Things to invite people to bring

- Drink
- Cushion/blanket to be comfortable
- Pen and paper for journalling
- Candle and matches

CIRCLE STORY: TESSA'S FORTIETH
BIRTHDAY GATHERING

As a circle holder, Tessa wanted a special celebration that brought her favourite people into a circle space. Given that it was a big gathering, there wasn't a talking element but different fun activities culminating with a ceremony facilitated by an experienced circle holder.

The event was held in a venue where she has taught yoga classes for years and runs workshops, so it feels very familiar and full of memories. It was a beautiful sunny day and people could spill out onto the lawn outside.

The first activity was learning a short belly dance fusion routine from her favourite dance teacher. People knew that this would be part of the gathering and came in comfortable clothing and gave it their best shot. This brought a sense of fun and lots of laughter with the upbeat Punjabi music.

Then they collected around a centrepiece with pebbles that had been painted with different uplifting words. A friend led some simple songs to bring a feeling of connection. It was only at this point that we realised that there was a power cut, because the electric piano didn't work, so she led the songs a cappella. Fortunately, the food didn't require heating and no-one wanted teas because it was such a hot day!

Then for the ceremony of abundance. The circle holder had set up a beautiful threshold with flowers. Each person was invited to move over the threshold in a way that felt authentic to them. Some walked serenely, others skipped, jumped, swirled or ran! It was funny and touching simultaneously. They were also invited to say a word to capture what they would like to have in abundance. Some kept the word to themselves; others shouted it out.

Finally, we sat around the centrepiece, and one by one each person chose a pebble with a word that had caught their eye, as a memento of the gathering. Then it was time for lunch and socialising.

Tessa shared:

Since the event, so many people have expressed that it was something really special to have a sense of ceremony as part of the gathering. For some of them, this was a completely new experience. For others, it was recognisable from their religious background, school rituals or from coming to the women's circle. I had given the theme of abundance to the circle holder and she came up with this beautiful idea of crossing the threshold. The years since have been abundant so we definitely manifested something that day.

Despite being very familiar with the venue and planning carefully, something unexpected still happened. When circle attendees have seen that you've planned and organised, an unexpected situation will bring you closer together.

When thinking about the logistics of running a circle, it can be easy to get bogged down in the details. However, they can contribute to creating a special experience. If you find yourself becoming overwhelmed, return to your intention for the circle: what is it that your gathering needs to function and what is on your wish list to make it even better later on?

We've seen so many people who intend to run a circle falter because they can't find the right venue. This can feel like a major barrier, but remember that the container you create for a gathering is only partly about the physical environment. If there is a need to come together, people will attend even if the venue is not perfect. The psychological container you create through the guidelines, structure of the circle and careful facilitation will be enough.

In the next chapter, we call on you to make a difference by being a circle holder. There are so many things that could stop us, and yet these special spaces for respectful listening and talking are so needed.

CHAPTER 20

A Call to Hold Circles

As we come to the end of this book, we want to encourage you in holding circle spaces in your community. Talking and listening circles can be transformational on a personal, community and global level. They are an ancient form of connection, starting in the simplest way: huddling around a fire. Circle gatherings can be simple and happen spontaneously. They can also be elaborate, with layers of ceremony.

The truth is there is no one right way of holding a circle space. We hope, though, that by giving you a structure, ideas about guidelines and different opening and closing practices, you will find a way to create a circle that feels authentic to you.

Sometimes people put barriers in their way to put off running the circle that they can see there is a need for or even that they know is their calling. These barriers might be finding the perfect venue, not being experienced enough or not knowing how to handle big emotions or how to market the circle. We invite you to just make a start because experience comes through doing.

Your circle may not be perfect the first time you run it, and you will tweak how you facilitate it over time. There may be a small number of people at the first one and that might be just the right number as you practise your circle holding skills. Maybe big emotions will come up during the gathering and you will respond as the compassionate human that you are.

If it feels like too big an undertaking to take on alone, speak to other like-minded people and see if you can collaborate. We are big fans of collaboration. We run circles together and love the support we can give each other. If one of us is not well, the other can take the session. If there is someone in our circle needing one-to-one support, one of us can dip out of the circle to support them. It also means we have ready-made emotional support as we can talk through how things went and how we feel about the circle once it is complete.

We take our self-care seriously. We both have listening partners, mentoring and circle support outside of the circles we run to give extra support. All of this eases the responsibility of facilitation. We recommend that you take whatever steps you need to ensure you have sufficient support to sustain you in this work. All the circle holders we spoke to had support networks around them to enable them to sustain their work.

We really believe that being in circle is in our blood, and yet many have not experienced being together and communicating in this way. In our research, we were surprised to hear from so many circle holders who had a profound experience in their thirties that had inspired them to take the brave step to set up spaces of their own and had not experienced circle previous to that. There were others who had been born into circle and have made it central to their lives as adults, and some who are still in their teenage years and are already on their path as circle holders.

If circle space was something used in schools with respectful listening and talking experienced from an early age, we wonder whether young people's mental health would improve. If circle events were held in work and community spaces, we're sure feelings of isolation would decrease. Running your circle matters.

A big thank you to all of the circle holders that we spoke to in the course of writing this book. The diversity, richness and creativity of gatherings was incredibly inspiring. Each facilitator we interviewed had started with one circle. They took the first step.

When you hold circles, you will find that you transform too. It's an honour and a privilege to create a container for people to share their authentic experiences. Seeking support to sustain and nourish yourself will enable you to be a circle holder for many years to come. As a facilitator, your capacity to hold big emotions and big topics will grow and we hope you will continue to do this humbly.

We love to hear from circle holders around the world.

Tell us where you are and who your circle is for.

Share why your circle means so much to you.

We also provide circle holding training. Do contact us if you would like to attend a workshop, training course or retreat.

Contact Julia: info@circleholding.org

Contact Tessa: tessa@tessavenutisanderson.co.uk

About the Authors

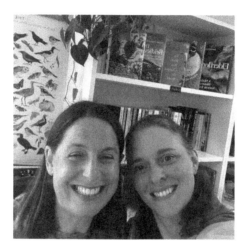

Julia and Tessa

Julia Davis

Julia hosts talking and listening circles both in person and online. She integrates circle holding into her yoga teacher training programmes and her yoga classes at Finchley Yoga studio. She runs circle-holding training both in person and online, including workshops, training courses and retreats and bespoke offerings. Her circle-holding skills originated in the youth groups she facilitated as a teenager.

She has taught yoga for over 20 years with specialisation in women's health therapy.

You can contact Julia at info@circleholding.org

www.circleholding.org

www.yogateachersforum.org

Tessa Venuti Sanderson

Tessa Venuti Sanderson founded her women's circle in 2014 and has since run a variety of circles, including mother and daughter, pregnancy and postnatal, menstrual cycle awareness, perimenopause and yoga teacher talking circles in person and online. Tessa runs circle facilitation training as well as yoga teacher CPD workshops. She is a yoga teacher specialising in women's health and birth trauma. Tessa mentors movement and body work professionals, and circle facilitators.

www.tessavenutisanderson.co.uk

Acknowledgements

Thank you to all of the circle holders who we have interviewed in the process of writing this book. You may wish to contact them to discover more about their circles.

Benedict Beaumont – www.makesomebreathingspace.com

Cecilia Allon – www.yogawithcecilia.co.uk

Daniel Groom – www.southendpride.org.uk and www.instagram.com/danielgroom_._

Gemma Brady – @sisterstoriesuk www.sisterstories.co

Henika Patel – https://schoolofsensualarts.co.uk

Israh Goodall – www.israhgoodall.com

Julia Paulette Hollenbery – https://universeofdeliciousness.com

Kate Codrington – www.katecodrington.co.uk

Lee Keylock – https://narrative4.com

Mark Walsh – https://embodimentunlimited.com

Sophie Cleere – www.instagram.com/sophie.cleere

Suzan Nolan and her Gather the Women circle – www.gatherthewomen.org

Tanya Forgan – https://tanyaforgan.com

Thank you to Anouska Ornstein, Matt Walker, Lisa Horwell, Mandy Lau, Barbara-Lee, Brenda Rock, Kate Forde, Joanna Feast, Alison Butler, Ariel Kahn, Lydia Martin, Mary Thorp, Frankie Culpin and Csilla Dulàcska.

Thank you also to all contributed their time but did not wish to be named.

With thanks also to:

www.alcoholics-anonymous.org.uk

https://samm.org.uk

Becoming Mums – https://becomingmums.com

Celebration Day for Girls – https://celebrationdayforgirls.com

Red School – www.redschool.net

Julia's acknowledgements

Thank you to family and friends who have listened to us talk about this book and held the fort while we have taken time away to write together. Particular thanks go to Adam, Zoe, Rosie, Edna and Barry Davis, Jill Shaw, Rachel Morris, Robert Shaw and Julie Bogush. Circle began for me in my community and with my family. Thank you for the many evenings sitting round the Friday night dinner table. Thank you to Louise and Hilton Nathanson for introducing us to circle table talk.

Thank you to everyone who has and continues to participate in and facilitate circles of all kinds at Finchley Yoga, including Melonie Syrett – our moon and drumming circles hold a special place in my heart. My experience of the local community is so much richer for the time I have spent in my happy place – I didn't realise just how special it was until the doors closed in March 2020 and I learned a whole new way of facilitating circle online.

Thank you to the teachers who I first gathered with before the teachers forum even had a name.

A huge thank you to everyone who has attended Yoga Teachers Forum over the years, from our inception in friends' houses, to my cottage studio and now all over the world! A special thank you to all my circle co-facilitators, including Aneta Idczak, Gabi Parkham, Jacqueline Rose, Jenni Stone and Fiona Agombar, for your support and encouragement.

Specific thanks to attendees of Yoga Nidra and Circle Holding Facilitator trainings. We loved sharing our ideas with you and thank you for all the feedback you have given us.

A special thank you to Tessa for trusting me when I asked you to co-create the labour of love that is this book.

In memory of Lucy, Maya and Rina Dee. May many families sit round the table together and ask the question 'What have you done for someone this week and what has someone done for you?'

Tessa's acknowledgements

A massive thank you to my family, Fabio, Zara and Alma, for supporting all my endeavours, even when it means I'll be away from home. I discovered the Red Tent through Uma Dinsmore-Tuli's book *Yoni Shakti* and from there Red School. Their workshops and retreats were the start of deep diving into understanding how to create space for supporting connection within circle time.

Thanks to all those women who've collaborated and held space with me, including Julia, Catherine Holt, Sophie Cleere and Barbara-Lee.

A tremendous thank you to all of the women that have attended the women's circle over the years at my home or in the yurt, who've seen my facilitation grow, many of whom now hold circles themselves. A special thanks to those who've supported the related books over the years and been cheerleaders for early versions.

So much gratitude towards the mothers who have brought their daughters to different circle gatherings and entrusted that I will guide their understanding of themselves and their bodies. I also appreciate all those people who have attended trainings that I have run, both on circle facilitation itself, and on all subjects, because you have helped me hone the way I want to create community and teach.

A last thank you to all of you who have gone on to run your own circle. These spaces are so needed to foster connection and respectful communication. I recognise your courage in taking a leap into the unknown and stepping up to be a leader in your community.

Thank you to everyone who has filled our lives with laughter, joy, tears and deep sharing from the heart in circle. This book is a celebration of all the possibilities that are created through circle.

Resources

References

Baldwin, Christina and Linnea, Ann (2010) *The Circle Way: A Leader in Every Chair*. Berrett-Koehler Publishers.

Emerson, David and Hopper, Elizabeth (2011) *Overcoming Trauma through Yoga: Reclaiming Your Body*. North Atlantic Books.

Gendlin, Eugene (1997) *Focusing*. Bantam Books

Kindred, Glennie (2003) *The Sacred Tree*. Self-published.

Kindred, Glennie (2013) *The Earth's Cycle of Celebration*. Wirksworth.

Orvell, Arianna, Kross, Ethan and Gelman, Susan (2017) How 'you' makes meaning. *Science* 355 (6331), 1299–1302.

Shafak, Elif (2016) *Three Daughters of Eve*. Viking Press (Kindle edition).

Teckentrup, Britta (2018) *Little Mouse and the Red Wall*. Orchard Books.

Other circle holding books

Shinoda Bolen, Jean (1999) *The Millionth Circle: How to Change Ourselves and the World: The Essential Guide to Women's Circles*. Conari.

Parker, Priya (2019) *The Art of Gathering: How We Meet and Why It Matters*. Penguin.

Florence, Anoushka (2022) *Women's Circle: How to Gather with Meaning, Intention and Purpose*. Quadrille Publishing.

Favourite books for circle readings

Foster, Jeff (2016) *The Way of Rest: Finding the Courage to Hold Everything in Love*. Sounds True Inc.

Lalla (1992) *Naked Song* (translated by Coleman Barks). Maypop Books.

O'Donohue, John (2007) *Benedictus*. Bantam Press.

Pinkola Estés, Clarissa (2008) *Women Who Run with Wolves: Contacting the Power of the Wild Woman*. Rider.

Roche, Lorin (2014) *The Radiance Sutras: 112 Gateways to the Yoga of Wonder and Delight*. Sounds True Inc.

Sampson, Ana (ed.) (2020) *She Is Fierce: Brave, Bold, and Beautiful Poems by Women*. Macmillan Children's Press.

Sieghart, William (2017) *The Poetry Pharmacy: Tried and True Prescriptions for the Heart, Mind and Soul*. Particular Books.

Teckentrup, Britta (2018) *Little Mouse and the Red Wall*. Orchard Books.

Teckentrup, Britta (2021) *When I See Red*. Prestel.

Children's resources

Guber, Tara and Fatus, Sophie (2005) *Yoga Pretzels: 50 Fun Activities for Kids and Grown Ups* (yoga cards). Abrams Books.

Innovative Resources: Online retailer which sells strength cards and bear cards to express emotions. https://innovativeresources.org/resources

Favourite oracle cards

Catling, Georgina. *Yoni Oracle Cards: Embody Your Lunar Nature.* https://goddesstemplegifts. co.uk/product/yoni-oracle-cards-created-by-georgina-catling

Dinsmore-Tuli, Uma and Tuli, Nirlipta. *Yoni Shakti Great Wisdom Goddess Temple Deck.* (Available at www.yoganidranetwork.org)

Gray, Kyle (2018) *Angels and Ancestors Oracle Cards.* Hay House.

Hillyer, Carolyn (2016). *Weavers' Oracle: Journey Cards and Travel Guide.* Seventh Wave Music. (Available at https://goddesstemplegifts.co.uk)

Other resources

Ann Weiser Cornell (2005) *The Radical Acceptance of Everything: Living a Focusing Life.* Callum Books. (Ann is a linguist and this book is very helpful on how to ask questions in a way that supports embodied enquiry.)